Ethik in den Biowissenschaften –
Sachstandsberichte des DRZE

Ethics in the Life Sciences –
DRZE Expert Reports

Band 21: Neuroenhancement

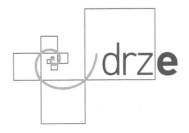

Commissioned by the
German Reference Centre for Ethics in the Life Sciences

Edited by
Dieter Sturma and Dirk Lanzerath

www.drze.de

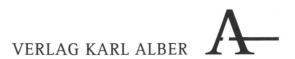

VERLAG KARL ALBER

Neuroenhancement concerns the improvement of a person's mental properties, abilities, and performance. These improvements can be achieved by diverse techniques and with different targets. Biochemical substances, medical devices, and behavioural strategies are employed in order to enhance, for example, cognition and mood.

The improvement of mental and physical properties, abilities, and performance has always been part of cultural history. The various techniques of neuroenhancement offer new opportunities of such improvement, but also come with substantive perils. Their employment may promote people's autonomy by facilitating self-expression. At the same time, however, these techniques may also undermine people's autonomy by making them the object of instrumentalization. Neuroenhancement thus involves significant normative challenges for individual persons as well as for society as a whole. In considering how neuroenhancement can be employed ethically, the benefits and risks must be carefully analysed.

This expert report provides a concise overview of the contemporary debate on neuroenhancement. It discusses the definition, techniques and targets of neuroenhancement and examines arguments for and against it at the level of individual persons, social interaction, and social policy.

Neuroenhancement hat die Verbesserung der mentalen Eigenschaften, Fähigkeiten und Leistung einer Person zum Gegenstand. Diese Verbesserungen können durch verschiedene Techniken und zu unterschiedlichen Zwecken erzielt werden. Biochemische Substanzen, medizinische Apparate und Verhaltensstrategien werden eingesetzt, um beispielsweise kognitive Prozesse zu optimieren und Stimmungen zu beeinflussen.

Die Verbesserung mentaler und physischer Eigenschaften, Fähigkeiten und Leistung war immer schon Teil der menschlichen Kulturgeschichte. Die verschiedenen Techniken des Neuroenhancement bieten neuartige Möglichkeiten der Verbesserung, bergen jedoch auch signifikante Gefahren. Sie können einerseits die Autonomie von Personen stärken, indem sie die Selbstentfaltung fördern. Andererseits kann die Autonomie von Personen durch den Einsatz dieser Techniken auch erheblich beeinträchtigt werden, wenn Personen zum Gegenstand von Instrumentalisierungen gemacht werden. Neuroenhancement stellt folglich sowohl Personen als auch die Gesellschaft im Ganzen vor umfassende normative Herausforderungen. Bei der Betrachtung, wie Neuroenhancement ethisch rechtfertigbar eingesetzt werden kann, müssen daher Nutzen und Risiken sorgfältig erwogen werden.

Der vorliegende Sachstandsbericht bietet einen konzisen Überblick über die gegenwärtige Neuroenhancement-Debatte. Definition, Techniken und Zwecke des Neuroenhancement werden erörtert und Argumente für und wider seine Anwendung auf personaler, interpersonaler sowie sozialpolitischer Ebene untersucht.

*Jan-Hendrik Heinrichs / Markus Rüther /
Mandy Stake / Julia Ihde*

Neuroenhancement

Verlag Karl Alber Baden-Baden

This publication is funded by the North Rhine-Westphalian Academy of Sciences, Humanities and the Arts as project of the Academy Program of the Federal Republic of Germany and the state of North Rhine-Westphalia.

The Deutsche Nationalbibliothek lists this publication in the Deutsche Nationalbibliografie; detailed bibliographic data are available on the Internet at http://dnb.d-nb.de
ISBN 978-3-495-49180-5 (Print)
        978-3-495-99961-5 (ePDF)

British Library Cataloging-in-Publication Data
A catalogue record for this book is available from the British Library.
ISBN 978-3-495-49180-5 (Print)
        978-3-495-99961-5 (ePDF)

Library of Congress Cataloging-in-Publication Data
Heinrichs, Jan-Hendrik | Rüther, Markus | Stake, Mandy | Ihde, Julia
Neuroenhancement
118 pp.
Includes bibliographic references and index.
ISBN 978-3-495-49180-5 (Print)
        978-3-495-99961-5 (ePDF)

Printed on acid-free paper

1st Edition 2022
© The Authors
Published by
VERLAG KARL ALBER –
a publishing company in the Nomos Verlagsgesellschaft, Baden-Baden 2022
Production of the printed version:
Nomos Verlagsgesellschaft mbH & Co. KG
Waldseestraße 3 – 5 | 76530 Baden-Baden
ISBN 978-3-495-49180-5 (Print)
eISBN 978-3-495-99961-5 (ePDF)

Contents

Contents

Preface

In a very general sense, enhancement is a process of improving the capabilities of a human person. Improvement can be achieved by invasive and non-invasive means or methods. Since the beginnings of human culture, persons have been transforming their environment and, in the process, also changed themselves. They have improved through language, technology, and organisation of the social space. In this context, *Bildung* and technical skills are constitutive sources of the improvement of the conditions for self-preservation and self-assertion of human individuals and societies. In contrast to other animal life forms, it is possible for individuals of the human life form to intentionally influence their capabilities. Historically, the technically and culturally improving human being has been the rule and by no means the exception.

Cultural improvements initially appear under the guise of technical impact on persons and their environment. As a result of scientific and technical progress, there has been a considerable expansion of direct influence on the physical and mental development of the human life form. This influence opens new scopes for action. In recent decades, technology-based enhancement has expanded significantly. This is mainly due to the availability of new invasive technical tools and pharmaceutical products. This form of improvement is now mostly referred to by the term ›enhancement‹. Unlike therapy, which is concerned with healing, reverting to a condition prior to illness, or reducing suffering, enhancement aims to improve a person's capabilities regardless of illness or suffering.

Recent methods of enhancement use performance-enhancing means and surgical or neurosurgical interventions to produce desired effects with less effort and, above all, in a shorter time compared with conventional practices. The desire for invasive performance enhancement often disguises constraints in personal life, school, university, and professional life that usually come about without the participation or consent of the persons concerned and are often neither attainable nor reasonable. Under these conditions, neuroenhancement amounts to surpassing requirements that are just about manageable by conventional means. Because the optimisations are pursued without a deeper understanding of the motives for the desire to improve performance and of the causes and reasons for the competitive relationships at play, they contribute to instrumentalization and self-instrumentalization.

The enhancement debate is ultimately based on two opposing conceptions of personal life. While cultural enhancement concerns a person who develops capabilities in a social space and interacts with her reality in initiatives and deliberate reactions, conceptions of invasive performance enhancement assume a passive person who transforms herself into desired states or allows herself to be put in those states, expecting a beneficial hedonistic outcome.

Due to the diversity of neurotechnical interventions, normative evaluations must relate directly to the respective fields of application. This applies to the distinction between therapy and enhancement as well as to the analysis of the relationship between disease and the consequences of intervention. For example, the evaluation of the use of deep brain stimulation in psychiatric disorders is fundamentally fraught with the difficulty that these interventions themselves have personality-altering effects. In this respect, the question of the consequences of intervention must be dealt with differently from that of the treatment of other dysfunctions. Also, the side effects of neurotechnical interventions and their long-term consequences are not yet well understood. Therefore, in each individual case, evaluations of the long-term effects must be balanced against the psychological and physical burdens imposed by the disease itself.

It may occur that changes in personality are considered problematic from a medical point of view or from the point of view of relatives but embraced by the patient. In a situation like this, the concept of authenticity is often invoked, but there are major epistemic obstacles when dealing with this concept. Practically, it is difficult to determine whether an expression of will can be considered authentic. This is true even for the corresponding subjective attitudes, which depend on relevant and comprehensible information and are embedded in specific social contexts. What makes it more difficult is that many applications of deep brain stimulation are or must be performed on patients whose capacity to understand and consent is limited due to the conditions of their disease.

The advocates of extensive enhancement in general and neuroenhancement in particular have the self-interest of individuals in mind. They see enhancement as a private endeavour rather than a social process. However, there have also been attempts to bring neuroenhancement and social justice into a direct relationship to compensate for social disadvantages in the development of personality and education as well as in the provision and redemption of life chances. Such compensations always bear the risk of instrumentalization due to the syndromes of self-deception and overattachment associated with neuroenhancement if they must be applied permanently. In this respect, neuroenhancement would aggravate the problem of social justice rather than compensate for inequality. To be sustainably anchored in a person's living conditions, justice must be realised socially—not technically.

Given the potentially far-reaching consequences for individual persons as well as for societies as a whole, neuroenhancement poses profound normative challenges. Possible dangers for individual persons and threats to the social framework must be considered. We must address the question how the techniques of neuroenhancement can be employed in ethically justifiable ways. For the time being, the search for answers will remain a source for debate and conflict.

This expert report provides a concise overview of the contemporary debate on neuroenhancement. It discusses the definition, techniques, and targets of neuroenhancement and examines arguments for and against it at the level of individual persons, social interaction, and social policy.

Dieter Sturma

I. Neuroenhancement – a short introduction on medical options

Julia Ihde

1.   Definition

In its broadest sense, the term ›neuroenhancement‹ refers to different types of measures taken by healthy people with the aim of increasing their performance, for example with regard to cognitive or emotional skills.[1] In contrast to the term ›enhancement‹, which also includes every kind of physical performance improvement (e.g. doping in sports), ›neuroenhancement‹ specifically refers to interventions that influence neurobiological processes in the brain. The focus of the discussion about neuroenhancement mostly lies on biochemical enhancement strategies, especially on the intake of pharmaceutical substances. Apart from that, there are many other ways to influence performance or behaviour, ranging from elements of daily life such as sleep or coffee consumption to physical measures such as brain stimulation. Although there are also considerations to influence other human behaviours such as moral behaviour,[2] targets of enhancement are primarily cognitive, motivational or emotional functions. This brief introduction will mainly focus on the enhancement of cognitive functions.[3]

---

[1] For a detailed overview of the definition of enhancement cf. section 4 (»What is enhancement? On the definition of enhancement«) of part 2 (Ethics of Neuroenhancement) of this expert report.

[2] For an example that covers this issue, cf. Sellaro et al. 2015. In this article, Sellaro et al. examined whether increasing cognitive control through brain stimulation helps overcome negative bias toward members of social out-groups.

[3] A short discussion of three targets of enhancement, cognition, mood and moral, is also provided in section 2 (»What can be enhanced? On the targets of (neuro-)enhancement«) of part 2 (Ethics of Neuroenhancement) of this expert report.

2. Possible targets of neuroenhancement and the measurability of its effects

The human mind consists of a broad variety of cognitive functions. Generally, cognitive performance is classified into different cognitive domains, which are again divided into subdomains.[4] The cognitive domains that are particularly interesting in the context of neuroenhancement are attention and concentration as well as memory which on their part have an impact on other, more complex domains such as executive functioning (e. g. reasoning and problem solving). There are no cognitive enhancers that augment every cognitive function in equal measures. Each enhancer or enhancing strategy, whether biochemical (e. g. pharmaceutical substances), behavioural (e. g. meditation or mnemonic strategies) or physical (e. g. brain stimulation), has a specific profile regarding its efficacy for different cognitive domains. For example, attention is enhanced by meditation, but not by mnemonic strategies. In contrast, memory can be enhanced through mnemonic strategies, but not by meditation.[5] Besides, there are cases where the enhancement of one domain by a certain enhancer goes along with the impairment of another cognitive domain. For example, methylphenidate, a prescription drug used to treat attention deficit hyperactivity disorder (ADHD), improves the ability to resist distraction, but impairs cognitive flexibility.[6]

The examination of different enhancement effects on cognitive functions relies on tests and methods used in clinical neuropsychology. Despite being designed to measure cognitive function in a standardised manner, there is a variety of neuropsychological test batteries. Studies show that the effects of pharmacological enhancement on different cognitive domains might differ depending on the cognitive test battery used.[7] Besides, not only the tests that are used might have an impact on the observable effects, but the effects are also influenced by personal factors, such as the cognitive skills of the individual prior to the enhancement intervention (the so-called *baseline performance*). Most pharmaceuticals

---

[4] There are different ways to conceptualise and organise cognitive ability domains. Cognitive functions can be classified either by the general process involved (e. g. attention, memory, or language), or by regional brain functions which are connected to certain cognitive functions, or in a hierarchy based on the complexion of the operations. Inconsistencies described in the clinical and research literature especially concern broad domains that may include multiple component processes. Cf. Harvey 2019: 227.

[5] Cf. Dresler et al. 2019: 1140.

[6] Cf. ibid., where they refer to Fallon et al. 2017.

[7] Cf. ibid., where they refer to Lees et al. 2017.

that are designed to treat conditions like dementia or ADHD primarily show their effects on individuals which have a low baseline performance, whereas for those subjects with a high baseline performance the pharmaceuticals show either no effect or can cause impairments of cognitive functions. This can be explained by the inverted U-model. It shows how optimal performances are achieved with intermediate levels of the targeted neurochemicals while impairments are caused by levels that are either too low or too high.[8] Basic biological and psychological factors, such as the genotype, gender, hormonal status, age or personality of a person[9], as well as social and socio-environmental factors, such as social resources, family composition or parental occupation, may also affect the efficiency of a cognitive enhancer.[10]

To sum up, the idea of a single pill or intervention improving all our cognitive skills at once and equally in every individual is not tenable. Every enhancer or enhancement strategy is targeted at a different set of cognitive functions and therefore influences different types of brain processes. Their efficiency depends on a variety of personal factors and may vary depending on the measurement method.

3.___Enhancement strategies

There are several ways of conceptualising the wide variety of enhancement strategies. For example, one can distinguish between pharmaceutical and non-pharmaceutical methods, between invasive and non-invasive methods, between psychopharmaceuticals / herbal medicine / dietary supplements and endogenous substances or between psychopharmaceuticals, neurostimulation and genetic manipulation.[11] In order to get the broadest possible overview of the different enhancement strategies, one can follow Martin Dresler et al. (2019) and differentiate between biochemical, physical and behavioural enhancement strategies.

---

[8] Cf. ibid. According to Dresler et al., a general baseline-dependency can also be observed in other enhancement strategies. In the cases of computer games, cognitive training or brain stimulation, individuals with a low baseline performance benefit more than individuals with a known high performance. Sleep, in contrast, rather improves memory functions for individuals with a previously detected higher baseline performance in memory or intelligence.

[9] A study by Smillie and Gökçen shows, for example, that caffeine enhances working memory especially in extraverted individuals. Cf. Smillie / Gökçen 2010 and Dresler et al. 2019: 1140.

[10] Cf. Dresler et al. 2019: 1140.

[11] Cf. also part 2 (Ethics of Neuroenhancement) of this expert report.

3.1   Biochemical strategies

3.1.1   Everyday substances and dietary supplements

There is a wide range of biochemical enhancement strategies. In the field of non-prescription daily substances, the widely socially accepted stimulants caffeine, taurine or glucose are most popular.[12] Numerous studies have shown that the consumption of sugar, coffee or other beverages from caffeine-bearing plants has cognition-enhancing effects.[13] In case of caffeine, for instance, its cognitive enhancing effects depend on the examination conditions. When information is learned passively, caffeine has performance-enhancing properties. However, this is not the case with regards to intentional learning. The substance can also increase the performance of working memory, but only if the level of difficulty is moderate; in complex tasks, caffeine even tends to reduce performance. Long-term memory does not seem to be affected by caffeine either. However, caffeine increases attention and vigilance and reduces response times; it develops its effects especially in sleep-deprived or exhausted subjects and also in repetitive cognitive tasks.[14] Other drugs that are typically used recreationally have also shown potential enhancement effects on cognition: nicotine might enhance attention;[15] alcohol, while impairing certain cognitive functions, might enhance creative processes.[16]

Additionally, there are numerous dietary supplements that promise positive effects on cognitive functions, e.g. preparations containing herbs like salvia,[17] *Bacopa monnieri* (in Indian herbal medicine known as brahmi),[18] ginseng or ginkgo biloba. So far, especially the last two have failed to show ascertainable positive effects on a range of targeted cognitive functions in healthy individuals.[19] Ginkgo biloba, for example, contains high concentrations of flavonoids and terpenoids, which were assumed to

---

[12] However, there are several controversial debates on possible health-damaging effects of these substances. Cf. for example Cappelletti 2015.

[13] Cf. Dresler et al. 2019: 1138, where they refer to Smith et al. 2011; Glade 2010 and Nehlig 2010.

[14] Cf. Gründer / Bartsch 2014: 1539.

[15] Cf. Dresler et al. 2019: 1139, where they refer to Warburton 1992 and Valentine / Sofuoglu 2018. Cf. also Gründer / Bartsch 2014: 1540.

[16] Cf. on this Jarosz / Colflesh / Wiley 2012 and Benedek et al. 2017.

[17] Cf. Dresler et al. 2019: 1138, who refer to Tildesley et al. 2003.

[18] Cf. Kongkeaw et al. 2014.

[19] Cf. Dresler et al. 2019: 1129, who refer to Laws / Sweetnam / Kondel 2012 and Geng et al. 2010.

counteract oxidative stress as antioxidants. However, according to a systematic literature review carried out by Andreas G. Franke and Klaus Lieb in 2010, gingko biloba showed no positive effects on reaction time and mood of healthy people and no consistent effects on vigilance, attention, memory, and subjective self-assessment.[20]

3.1.2 (Psycho-)Pharmaceuticals

Much of the discussion about neuroenhancement revolves around the use of drugs that were designed to treat conditions such as dementia, ADHD or depression. In the media, medications that are used off-label to improve cognition are often referred to as ›intelligent drugs‹. For various reasons, determining how broadly intelligent drugs are used is only possible to a limited extent. Results might vary depending on the definition of neuroenhancement, heterogeneous investigation populations or the type of investigation (samplings, tolls etc.). Although determining the prevalence of illegal substances and medication used for enhancing purposes is linked to certain difficulties, there have been tolls and surveys examining how widespread biochemical neuroenhancement strategies are.[21] Since 2009, there have been three representative surveys on neuroenhancement in Germany carried out by the Robert Koch Institute and the Deutsche Angestellten-Krankenkasse (German employee health insurance, DAK).[22] According to the population-based study (Studie zum Konsum leistungsbeeinflussender Mittel in Alltag und Freizeit, KOLIBRI) by the Robert Koch Institute in 2010, 1.5% of the German population used medication without medical indications or illegal substances for enhancement purposes.[23] The study also reveals that younger people and people with high weekly working hours are more likely to take intelligent drugs.[24] In 2009 and 2015, the DAK conducted online surveys on 3,000 and 5,000 DAK insured persons. The evaluation of the online surveys shows that about 5% (2009) and 6.7% (2015) of employees between the ages of 20 and 50 take medication or other substances for enhancement purposes without medical indications. In their second study from 2015,

---

[20] Cf. Franke / Lieb 2010: 858.
[21] The discussion was mainly initiated by a poll carried out by *Nature* magazine in 2008, cf. for this Maher 2008.
[22] Cf. Müller / Freude / Kersten 2019.
[23] Cf. Schilling et al. 2012: 2.
[24] The usage of substances like methylphenidate seems to be especially high among students. Cf. on this Carton et al. 2018 and Cândido et al. 2019.

they conclude that especially employees with simple or insecure jobs belong to the risk groups for medication abuse linked to enhancement.[25]

Especially D-amphetamine and methylphenidate have well documented cognitive-enhancing properties in healthy test subjects.[26] Amphetamines and methylphenidate, both used to treat ADHD,[27] block presynaptic norepinephrine and dopamine transporters. As a result, they increase monoaminergic neurotransmission due to a lack of negative feedback.[28] Amphetamine is known for increasing long-term attention, counteracting the reduction of performance after sleep deprivation and overall reducing the need for sleep.[29] A review of single dose studies conducted by Anke Linssen et al. (2014) comes to the conclusion that methylphenidate improves cognitive performance especially in the domains of working memory and speed of processing; to a lesser extent it may also improve verbal learning and memory, attention and vigilance as well as reasoning and problem solving.[30] However, according to Dresler et al., the empirical evidence for the efficacy of synthetic stimulants for enhancing brain function and cognition in healthy subjects is often markedly lower than assumed in theoretical discussion. As mentioned before, the effects of methylphenidate and other synthetic stimulants are not only baseline-dependent, but placebo effects must be considered as well.[31]

Another drug that is considered as potential neuroenhancer is modafinil, a medication originally used to treat sleepiness due to narcolepsy, shift work sleep disorder, or obstructive sleep apnoea; depression in bipolar disorder, fatigue syndrome in depression and ADHD are also examined as further potential indications.[32] The exact therapeutic effect mechanism of modafinil is still unknown. However, studies have shown that it induces an increase in various monoamines such as dopamine, noradrenaline and serotonin. It was also proven that modafinil causes a histamine release into the central nervous system, which promotes vigilance. Yet, its effectiveness as a neuroenhancer in healthy, non-sleep-deprived subjects remains controversial among experts. A meta-analysis by Ruair-

---

[25] Cf. Deutsche Angestellten-Krankenkasse 2009; id. 2015.
[26] Cf. Gründer / Bartsch 2014: 1540.
[27] Under German law, amphetamines, which are an approved medication to treat ADHD in the US, are classified as illegal substances. In Germany, mainly methylphenidate, best known under its trading name Ritalin, is used for the treatment of ADHD and less frequently for narcolepsy.
[28] Cf. Franke / Lieb 2010: 854.
[29] Cf. Gründer / Bartsch 2014: 1539.
[30] Cf. Linssen 2014: 973.
[31] Cf. for example Cropsey et al. 2017.
[32] Cf. Förstl 2009: 843.

idh Battleday and Anna-Katharine Brem (2015) concluded that modafinil has genuine cognitive enhancing effects on some cognitive domains without causing severe side effects or changes in mood. In studies that used complex assessments, modafinil appears to improve attention, executive functions and learning consistently. In contrast, only half of the studies included in the meta-analysis that used basic testing paradigms came to similar results.[33] Zackary Cope et al. (2017) also describe modafinil as an effective cognitive enhancer in healthy adult subjects. Compared to other stimulants, the cognitive enhancing effect is achieved at doses that do not result in hyperactivity.[34] In this sense, one can conclude that it acts similarly to methylphenidate, nevertheless, without the adverse side effects of the amphetamine-like substances.[35] In addition, studies indicate that no substantial baseline-dependent effects appear to be caused.[36]

Antidementia drugs, such as acetylcholinesterase inhibitors and memantine, are also considered to initiate cognitive enhancing effects in healthy subjects. So far, only few studies exist on the issue. Most of them examine the medication donepezil.[37] Donepezil is a potent acetylcholinesterase inhibitor; by blocking the acetylcholinesterase, the enzymatic breakdown of acetylcholine in the synaptic cleft is inhibited and the concentration of acetylcholine in the synaptic cleft is increased.[38] In subjects suffering from dementia, this appears to reduce symptoms of the disease. However, a meta-analysis by Dimitris Repantis et al. (2010) on acetylcholinesterase inhibitors and memantine for neuroenhancement in healthy individuals indicates that there is no consistent evidence for a cognitive enhancing effect of donepezil in healthy people. According to six small trials, donepezil might improve the retention of training on complex aviation tasks and verbal memory for semantically processed words. Nevertheless, results were especially inconsistent regarding positive effects on episodic memory.[39] A reduction of memory and attention deficits was only observed in subjects with a 24-hour sleep deprivation but not in rested individuals.[40]

---

[33] Cf. on this Battleday / Brem 2015.
[34] Cf. on this Cope et al. 2017.
[35] Cf. Förstl 2009: 843.
[36] Cf. d'Angelo / Savulich / Sahakian 2017: 3260.
[37] Cf. ibid.
[38] Cf. Brewster et al. 2019: 159.
[39] Cf. d'Angelo / Savulich / Sahakian 2017: 3260, who refer to Repantis / Laisney / Heuser 2010.
[40] Cf. Repantis / Laisney / Heuser 2010, who refer to Chuah / Chee 2008.

3.1.3 ›Microdosing‹

Besides the use of widespread illegal substances that are not only taken for recreational, but also for performance enhancing purposes—e. g. amphetamines (speed or crystal meth), cocaine and novel psychoactive substances (NPS, also called designer drugs)—, a trend has emerged in recent years which promotes the intake of minimal doses of mostly illegal psychedelic substances, referred to as microdosing. The idea behind this is that the regular ingestion of very small quantities of psychedelic substances like lysergic acid diethylamide (LSD) and psilocybin might lead to mental health benefits such as an improvement of creativity and attention and a reduction of depression and anxiety. Research on psychedelics has been performed for decades and despite highly controversial debates, it provides evidence for therapeutic effects of full-doses.[41] In contrast, since microdosing is quite a young phenomenon there is barely any empirical research. Vince Polito and Richard J. Stevenson (2019) have summarised the results of the four scientific articles on microdosing existing to date.[42] Three of them, describing qualitative interview studies and observational studies, report positive outcomes, namely an improvement of mood, energy levels and cognition, open-mindedness and creativity as well as a reduction of negative attitudes and emotions.[43] These results are based on interviews or small-scale non-blinded, non-placebo-controlled experiments; one must assume that there are significant placebo effects. The only randomised, double-blind, placebo-controlled trial on LSD microdosing by Steliana Yanakieva et al. (2019) concludes that microdosing LSD can lead to changes in time perception. However, benefits on health, cognition or well-being were not investigated.[44] In summary, in view of promising results of existing research on full-dose psychedelics it has yet to be shown whether small doses of psychedelics could have cognitive enhancing effects. Further empirical research is required to determine the effectiveness of microdosing.

3.1.4 Genetic editing

For some years, a new generation of genetic engineering techniques, including CRISPR-Cas9, has been revolutionising the whole field of genetic editing, promising more precise, more effective and more economic

---

[41] Cf. Prochazkova et al. 2018: 3402–3403; Anderson et al. 2019: 732.
[42] Cf. Polito / Stevenson 2019.
[43] Cf. Johnstad 2018; Prochazkova et al. 2018 and Anderson et al. 2019.
[44] Cf. Yanakieva et al. 2019.

interventions in the human genome.[45] These innovations have made the once seemingly distant, unrealistic idea of improving cognitive performance through genetic engineering more probable. However, apart from the ethical problems that would accompany such interventions, this research area is still in its early days. So far, the question of which cognitive functions are influenced by which gene expressions has been the subject of basic research. The idea of cognitive enhancement through genetic editing is thus only subject of hypothetical considerations. An article by Andrea Lavazza (2018) examines the possibilities and critical issues related to enhancement via genetic engineering.[46] He describes certain difficulties besides ethical issues that arise in this context. Although it is a well-established belief that genes are not only the basis of inheritable traits but also of cognitive abilities, the idea of one gene or a small set of genes that can be identified with a certain cognitive function might be misleading. Although certain cognitive functions can be linked to a single gene or a small group of genes, complex brain processes do not seem to depend on these alone. The main cognitive functions involve different brain areas and probably a cascade of neuronal activations which requires the expression of many genes.[47] Besides, research on complex epigenetic mechanisms shows that the expression of genes also depends on their interaction with the development and on the external environment of the individual.[48]

In addition to the fact that it is difficult or maybe even impossible to discover a specific gene (or a small set of genes) that is responsible for a specific cognitive function, there are certain risks regarding the insertion of modified gene sequences into the cells of the human body. In gene therapy, mainly viruses are used as vectors to deliver genetic material into cells. This technique bears several risks, for example, the risk of an immune reaction or the incorrect integration of the modified genetic material into the genome. Although techniques like CRISPR-Cas9 appear to be more accurate, the risk of incorrect gene-cuts or inaccurate insertion events remains. Moreover, for cognitive enhancement, vectors or other insertion techniques would have to traverse the blood-brain barrier to reach the neurons where the target genes are mainly expressed.[49]

---

[45] First described by Doudna / Charpentier 2014.
[46] Cf. Lavazza 2018.
[47] Cf. ibid.: 390.
[48] Cf. ibid. Lavazza refers to Bonduriansky / Day 2018.
[49] Cf. ibid.: 389.

In order to get from hypothetical considerations to actual possible applications, significant amount of research is still required, which can only be partly justified to this date. Considering the current state of knowledge about gene therapy, experimental applications of genetic editing should only be authorised on patients likely to pass away due to a severe disease that cannot be treated otherwise or on patients suffering from other serious diseases. Since genetic editing techniques intervene in complex processes that are not yet completely understood, modifying the expression of one gene could lead to unwanted, serious, and irreversible effects. Accordingly, non-clinical applications of new gene editing techniques can currently be ruled out because of general safety issues.[50]

3.2   Physical strategies

3.2.1   Brain stimulation

In the field of physical enhancement strategies, especially brain stimulation techniques are discussed regarding their potential cognitive enhancement effects on healthy subjects. Brain stimulation techniques have been developed for therapeutic purposes in psychiatry and neurology. Today they are used to treat conditions such as Parkinson's disease, epilepsy, chronic pain, or major depression. Some of these methods also show enhancing effects on the cognition of healthy individuals.[51] A distinction is generally made between two main types of brain stimulation: invasive and non-invasive methods.

Deep brain stimulation (DBS) is an invasive brain stimulation technique. It requires a neurosurgical procedure, during which a medical device —a neurostimulator which sends electrical impulses (also called *brain pacemaker*)—is placed inside the brain. It is considered as a promising treatment for a variety of neurological and psychiatric conditions.[52] Besides, studies have shown that DBS might enhance the memory of patients with intractable epilepsy.[53] However, since it requires a neurosurgical procedure and is, therefore, associated with a risk that is not proportionate without medical indication, it is restricted to subjects with pathological conditions.

---

[50] Cf. Lavazza 2018: 391.
[51] Cf. Dresler et al. 2013: 535. Cf. also McKinley et al. 2011.
[52] Cf. Aum / Tierney 2018.
[53] Cf. Inman et al. 2018 and Suthana et al. 2012.

There are also several non-invasive methods that are associated with rather low risks and minor side effects, for example electrical stimulation methods such as transcranial direct current stimulation (tDCS), transcranial alternating current stimulation (tACS), transcranial random noise stimulation (tRNS), transcranial pulsed current stimulation (tPCS), or transcutaneous vagus nerve stimulation (tVNS).[54] In the case of these non-invasive electric stimulation methods, usually electrodes that are connected with a battery-powered device are placed on the head. This enables the stimulation of the human brain using electrical impulses. There are other, similar methods that work with magnetic impulses (e.g. transcranial magnetic stimulation, TMS). Those methods use a magnetic coil that is applied tangentially to the skull and creates a short magnetic field. Either way, brain activity is influenced by modulating the membrane potential to provoke cognitive, emotional, and behavioural changes. The stimulation is intended to increase or inhibit the activity, connectivity and sensitivity of nerve cells. These techniques are, for instance, used in research. In combination with imaging methods, they allow an investigation into causal relationships between brain areas and behaviour. A small number of them are also used in clinical practice (mostly tDCS and TMS).[55] However, recent studies have questioned whether some of the commonly used techniques (like tDCS) have neurophysiologically meaningful effects at all.[56] Although there are a number of studies that suggest enhancing effects on cognitive functions such as memory and learning,[57] it is impossible to assume that brain stimulation methods in general have clear and simple enhancing effects.[58] Thus, their efficacy strongly depends on applying the devices and electrodes to the correct region; individual variation in anatomy and response often occurs.[59] Another problem concerns the clear identification of brain areas and cognitive functions. To achieve a response linked to certain cognitive skills, it is crucial to understand which area must be stimulated. This area of research must be further investigated.[60] Besides electrical and magnetic stimulation methods, techni-

---

[54] Cf. Dresler et al. 2019: 1139. Transcranial means ›through the skull (cranium)‹; transcutaneous ›through the skin (cutis)‹.
[55] Cf. Science Media Center Germany 2019.
[56] Cf. Dresler et al. 2019: 1139, who refer to Lafon et al. 2017; Thibaut et al. 2017; Parkin et al. 2018 and Grossman et al. 2017.
[57] Cf. Dresler et al. 2013: 536.
[58] Cf. Dresler et al. 2019: 1139.
[59] Cf. Dresler et al. 2013: 536.
[60] Cf. ibid: 536.

ques that use optical stimulation via lasers or acoustic stimulation[61] are also assumed to have a potential for cognitive enhancement.

3.2.2 Biohacking devices

In recent years, a new debate on physical tools that assist cognitive functioning arose in the context of biohacking communities. The term ›biohacking‹ describes a do-it-yourself citizen science that merges body modification with technology. Although this community of hobbyist software developers is primarily interested in tracking their daily physical and biochemical activities in order to maintain a healthy lifestyle based on the data they gain, there are also attempts to create devices that enhance cognitive functions directly.[62] These include technical devices such as wearable electronic memory aids, augmented reality gadgets or neural implants that—under controlled laboratory settings—showed enhancing effects on human memory.[63] However, do-it-yourself enhancement methods bear specific risks that should not be underestimated. In this context, clear regulations must yet be determined.

3.3 *Behavioural strategies*

In addition to biochemical and physical methods, there are methods and activities belonging to our everyday or cultural activities that help improve certain cognitive skills. These include sleep, physical exercise, learning a second language as well as meditation, computerized training, or mnemonic techniques.

3.3.1 Sleep

The neural mechanisms underlying the effects of sleep on cognitive functions like memory consolidation are not yet completely understood. However, research literature suggests that enhancing cognitive functions, especially memory and creativity, is one important function of sleep.[64] Accordingly, sleep deprivation impairs neurocognitive functioning, parti-

---

[61] Cf. Dresler et al. 2019: 1139.
[62] Cf. Yetisen 2018: 744.
[63] Cf. Dresler et al. 2019: 1139, who refer i. a. to Warwick 2014 and Hampson et al. 2018.
[64] Cf. Dresler et al. 2013: 532, who refer to Diekelmann / Born 2010. On the effects of sleep on memory consolidation also cf. Chambers 2017.

cularly within the domains of sustained attention and executive function. At the same time, there are studies that suggest that the neurocognitive effects of sleep restriction are differentially tolerated by different age groups. Elderly subjects are affected more than younger adult subjects.[65]

3.3.2 Physical exercise

It is well known that regular physical activity helps to stay healthy in general. Furthermore, there is evidence suggesting that regular aerobic exercise has beneficial effects on brain functions and cognition.[66] A meta-analysis of randomised controlled trials by Patrick J. Smith et al. (2010) concluded that aerobic exercise training enhances attention, processing speed and executive function.[67] Although data on the neural mechanism underlying the effects of physical exercise on human cognition is still relatively sparse, there is sufficient evidence that physical exercise enhances cognitive functions throughout the lifespan.[68]

3.3.3 Cultural activities

Several studies have shown that music training has a broad range of positive effects on cognition. Playing an instrument requires constant training of highly specialised sensorimotor, auditory, and auditory-spatial skills. It was observed that the brains of people who play an instrument differ from those who do not. This leads to the question if music training or pre-existing biological dispositions for musicality are responsible for this difference. A meta-analysis by Assal Habibi et al. (2018) concludes that music training induces brain and behavioural changes in children, which are not attributable to pre-existing biological traits.[69] In addition, music training also shows cognition enhancing effects on older adults. Sofia Seinfeld et al. (2013) describe a significant improvement of executive functions, inhibitory control and divided attention, a trend indicating an enhancement of visual scanning and motor ability and finally a decrease of depression and an evocation of positive mood states linked to regular

---

[65] Cf. Lowe / Safati / Hall 2017: 600.
[66] Cf. Dresler et al. 2013: 532, who refer to Hillman / Erickson / Kramer 2008.
[67] Cf. Smith et al. 2010. For other meta-analyses on cognition enhancing effects of physical exercise that come to similar results cf. Chang et al. 2012; Roig et al. 2013 and Hötting / Röder 2013.
[68] Cf. Dresler et al. 2013: 532.
[69] Cf. Habibi et al. 2018.

piano lessons given to older adults.[70] Besides instrumental training, learning a second language similarly shows enhancing effects. For example, a study by Ellen Bialystok, Fergus I. M. Craik and Gigi Luk (2012) concludes that bilingualism might protect against cognitive decline in older age.[71] And even contemporary dance improvisation might be a useful way to improve cognitive flexibility in aging. A study by Olivier A. Coubard et al. (2011), for example, suggests that high attentional dance improvisation improves switching attention in older adults.[72]

3.3.4 Cognitive training techniques

There are several training techniques such as mnemonic techniques or meditation that have been developed and used for centuries to enhance certain cognitive functions. Mnemonic training might lead to superior memory performance[73] while meditation training enhances attention processes and mindfulness.[74] While these results are widely accepted, the effects of computerised training and commercial computer games are rather controversial. There are concerns that especially violent computer games might have a negative impact on social behaviour, leading to an increase of aggression and reduction of empathy.[75] However, there is a growing interest in computerised training programs that are designed to enhance long term memory or brain plasticity in healthy or mildly impaired older adults to prevent conditions such as dementia.[76] However, recent studies give rise to doubt concerning the efficacy of computer training programs and the transferability of their positive effects on cognitive skills outside the computer game or training program.[77]

In contrast to biochemical or physical enhancement strategies, behavioural methods are hardly ever linked to health risks and ethical concerns. In some cases, their impact on human cognition seems to be greater than the impact of pharmaceutical or physical interventions. In addition, they are easily accessible to a large majority of people, for example in the case

---

[70] Cf. Seinfeld et al. 2013.
[71] Cf. Bialystok / Craik / Luk 2012.
[72] Cf. Coubard et al. 2011.
[73] Cf. Dresler et al. 2017.
[74] Cf. Dresler et al. 2019: 1139, who refer to Chiesa / Calati / Serretti 2011 and Sedlmeier et al. 2012.
[75] Cf. Dresler et al. 2013: 535, who refer to Kirsh / Mounts 2007 and Anderson et al. 2010.
[76] Cf. Dresler et al. 2013: 535, who refer to Tardif / Simard 2011. Also cf. Hill et al. 2017.
[77] Cf. Dresler et al. 2019: 1139, who refer to Simons et al. 2016; Melby-Lervåg / Redick / Hulme 2016 and Stojanoski et al. 2018.

of physical exercise and meditation. However, they are time-consuming, which is why research on more efficient means of improving human performance will certainly continue to be conducted.

References

Anderson, C. A. / Shibuya, A. / Ihori, N. / Swing, E. L. / Bushman, B. J. / Sakamoto, A. / Rothstein, H. R. / Saleem, M. (2010): Violent video game effects on aggression, empathy, and prosocial behavior in eastern and western countries: a meta-analytic review. In: Psychological Bulletin, 136 (2), 151–173.

Anderson, T. / Petranker, R. / Dinh-Williams, L.-A. / Rosenbaum, D. / Weissman, C. / Hapke, E. / Farb, N. A. S. (2019): Microdosing Psychedelics: Personality, mental health, and creativity differences in microdosers. In: Pharmacology 236, 731–740.

d'Angelo, L. C. / Savulich, G. / Sahakian, B. J. (2017): Lifestyle use of drugs by healthy people for enhancing cognition, creativity, motivation and pleasure. In: British Journal of Pharmacology 174, 3257–3267.

Aum, D. J. / Tierney, T. S. (2018): Deep brain stimulation: foundations and future trends. In: Frontiers in Bioscience 23, 162–182.

Battleday, R. M. / Brem, A.-K. (2015): Modafinil for cognitive neuroenhancement in healthy non-sleep-deprived subjects: A systematic review. In: European Neuropsychopharmacology 25 (11), 1865–1881.

Benedek, M. / Panzierer, L. / Jauk, E. / Neubauer, A. C. (2017): Creativity on tap? Effects of alcohol intoxication on creative cognition. In: Consciousness and Cognition 56, 128–134.

Bialystok, F. / Craik, F. I. M. / Luk, G. (2012): Bilingualism: Consequences for mind and brain. In: Trends in Cognitive Sciences 16 (4), 240–250.

Bonduriansky, R. / Day, T. (2018): Extended Heredity: A New Understanding of Inheritance and Evolution. Princeton: Princeton University Press.

Brewster, J. T. / Dell'Acqua, S. / Thach, D. Q. / Sessler, J. L. (2019): Classics in Chemical Neuroscience: Donepezil. In: ACS Chemical Neuroscience 10 (1), 155–167.

Cândido, R. C. F. / Perini, E. / Pádua, C. M. / Junqueira, D. R. (2019): Prevalence of and factors associated with the use of methylphenidate for cognitive enhancement among university students. In: Einstein (Sao Paulo), eAO4745.

Cappelletti, S. / Piacentino, D. / Sani, G. / Aromatario, M. (2015): Caffeine: Cognitive and Physical Performance Enhancer or Psychoactive Drug? In: Current Neuropharmacology 13, 71–88.

Carton, L. / Cabé, N. / Ménard, O. / Deheul, S. / Caous, A.-S. / Devos, D. / Cottencin, O. / Bordet, R. (2018): Pharmaceutical cognitive doping in students: A chimeric way to get-a-head? In: Therapies 73 (4), 331–339.

Chambers, A. M. (2017): The role of sleep in cognitive processing: focusing on memory consolidation. In: Wires Cognitive Science 8 (3), e1433.

Chang, Y. K. / Labban, J. D. / Gapin, J. I. / Etnier, J. L. (2012): The effects of acute exercise on cognitive performance: a meta-analysis. In: Brain Research 1453, 87–101.

Chiesa, A. / Calati, R. / Serretti, A. (2011): Does mindfulness training improve cognitive abilities? A systematic review of neuropsychological findings. In: Clinical Psychology Review 31 (3), 449–464.

Chuah L. Y. / Chee, M. W. (2008): Cholinergic augmentation modulates visual task performance in sleep-deprived young adults. In: The Journal of Neuroscience 28 (44), 11369–11377.

Cope, Z. A. / Minassian, A. / MacQueen, D. A. / Milienne-Periot, M. / Geyer, M. A. / Perry, W. / Young, J. W. (2017): Modafinil improves attentional performance in healthy, non-sleep deprived humans at doses not inducing hyperarousal across species. In: Neuropharmacology 125, 254–262.

Coubard, O. A. / Duretz, S. / Lefebvre, V. / Lapalus, P. / Ferrufino, L. (2011): Practice of contemporary dance improves cognitive flexibility in aging. In: Frontiers in Aging Neuroscience 3, 13.

Cropsey, K. L. / Schiavon, S. / Hendricks, P. S. / Froelich, M. / Lentowicz, I. / Fargason, R. (2017): Mixed-amphetamine salts expectancies among college students: Is stimulant induced cognitive enhancement a placebo effect? In: Drug and Alcohol Dependence 178, 302–309.

Deutsche Angestellten Krankenkasse (ed.) (2009): Gesundheitsreport 2009. Analyse der Arbeitsunfähigkeitsdaten. Schwerpunktthema Doping am Arbeitsplatz. Hamburg: DAK.

Deutsche Angestellten Krankenkasse (ed.) (2015): DAK-Gesundheitsreport 2015. Hamburg: DAK.

Diekelmann, S. / Born, J. (2010): The memory function of sleep. In: Nature Reviews Neuroscience 11, 114–126.

Doudna, J. A. / Charpentier, E. (2014): The new frontier of genome engineering with CRISPR-Cas9. In: Science 346 (6213), 1258096.

Dresler, M. / Sandberg, A. / Ohla, K. / Bublitz, C. / Trenado, C. / Mroczko-Wąsowicz, A. / Kühn, S. / Repantis, D. (2013): Non-pharmacological cognitive enhancement. In: Neuropharmacology 64, 529–543.

Dresler, M. / Shirer, W. R. / Konrad, B. N. / Müller, N. C. J. / Wagner, I. C. / Fernández, G. / Czisch, M. / Greicius, M. D. (2017): Mnemonic training reshapes brain networks to support superior memory. In: Neuron 93 (5), 1227–1235.e6.

Dresler, M. / Sandberg, A. / Bublitz, C. / Ohla, K. / Trenado, C. / Mroczko-Wąsowicz, A. / Kühn, S. / Repantis, D. (2019): Hacking the Brain: Dimensions of Cognitive Enhancement. In: ACS Chemical Neuroscience 19, 1137–1148.

Fallon, S. J. / van der Schaaf, M. E. / Ter Huurne, N. / Cools, R. (2017): The Neurocognitive Cost of Enhancing Cognition with Methylphenidate: Improved Distractor Resistance but Impaired Updating. In: Journal of Cognitive Neuroscience 29 (4), 652–663.

Förstl, H. (2009): Neuro-Enhancement. Gehirndoping. In: Nervenarzt 80, 840–846.

Franke, A. G. / Lieb, K. (2010): Pharmakologisches Neuroenhancement und »Hirndoping«. Chancen und Risiken. In: Bundesgesundheitsblatt 53, 853–860.

Geng, J. / Dong, J. / Ni, H. / Lee, M. S. / Wu, T. / Jiang, K. / Wang, G. / Zhou, A. L. / Malouf, R. (2010): Ginseng for cognition. In: Cochrane Database of Systematic Reviews 12, CD007769.

Glade, M. J. (2010): Caffeine—Not just a stimulant. In: Nutrition 26 (10), 932–938.

Grossman, N. / Bono, D. / Dedic, N. / Kodandaramaiah, S. B. / Rudenko, A. / Suk, H. J. / Cassara, A. M. / Neufeld, E. / Kuster, N. / Tsai, L. H. / Pascual-Leone, A. / Boyden, E. S. (2017): Noninvasive Deep Brain Stimulation via Temporally Interfering Electric Fields. In: Cell 169, 1029.

Gründer, G. / Bartsch, T. (2014): Neuroenhancement. In: Nervenarzt 85, 1536–1543.

Habibi, A. / Damasio, A. / Ilari, B. / Sachs, M. E. / Damasio, H. (2018): Music training and child development: a review of recent findings from longitudinal study. In: Annals of the New York Academy of Sciences 1423, 73–81.

Hampson, R. E. / Song, D. / Robinson, B. S. / Fetterhoff, D. / Dakos, A. S. / Roeder, B. M. / She, X. / Wicks, R. T. / Witcher, M. R. / Couture, D. E. / Laxton, A. W. / Munger-Clary, H. / Popli, G. / Sollman, M. J. / Whitlow, C. T. / Marmarelis, V. Z. / Berger, T. W. / Deadwyler, S. A. (2018): Developing a hippocampal neural prosthetic to facilitate human memory encoding and recall. In: Journal of Neural Engineering 15 (3), 036014.

Harvey, P. D. (2019): Domains of cognition and their assessment, In: Dialogues in Clinical Neuroscience 21 (3), 227–237.

Hill, N. T. M. / Mowszowski, L. / Naismith, S. L. / Chadwick, V. L. / Valenzuela, M. / Lampit, A. (2017): Computerized cognitive training in older adults with mild cognitive impairment or dementia: A systematic review and meta-analysis. In: The American Journal of Psychiatry 174 (4), 329–340.

Hillman, C. H. / Erickson, K. I. / Kramer, A. F. (2008): Be smart, exercise your heart: exercise effects on brain and cognition. In: Nature Reviews Neuroscience 9, 58–65.

Hötting, K. / Röder, B. (2013): Beneficial effects of physical exercise on neuroplasticity and cognition. In: Neuroscience & Biobehavioral Reviews 37 (8), 2243–2257.

Inman, C. S. / Manns, J. R. / Bijanki, K. R. / Bass, D. I. / Hamann, S. / Drane, D. L. / Fasano, R. E. / Kovach, C. K. / Gross, R. E. / Willie, J. T. (2018): Direct electrical stimulation of the amygdala enhances declarative memory in humans. In: PNAS 115 (1), 93–103.

Jarosz, A. F. / Colflesh, G. J. / Wiley, J. (2012): Uncorking the muse: alcohol intoxication facilitates creative problem solving. In: Consciousness and Cognition 21 (1), 487–493.

Johnstad, P. G. (2018): Powerful substances in tiny amounts: An interview study of psychedelic microdosing. In: Nordic Studies on Alcohol and Drugs 35, 39–51.

Kirsh, S. J. / Mounts, J. R. W. (2007): Violent video game play impacts facial emotion recognition. In: Aggressive Behavios 33 (4), 353–358.

Kongkeaw, C. / Dilokthornsakul, P. / Thanarangsarit, P. / Limpeanchob, N. / Norman Scholfield, C. (2014): Meta-analysis of randomized controlled trials on cognitive effects of Bacopa monnieri extract. In: Journal of Ethnopharmacology 151 (1), 528–535.

Lafon, B. / Henin, S. / Huang, Y. / Friedman, D. / Melloni, L. / Thesen, T. / Doyle, W. / Buzsaki, G. / Devinsky, O. / Parra, L. C. / Liu, A. A. (2017): Low frequency transcranial electrical stimulation does not entrain sleep rhythms measured by human intracranial recordings. In: Nature Communications 8, 1199.

Lavazza, A. (2018): Cognitive Enhancement through Genetic Editing: a New Frontier to explore (and to regulate)? In: Journal of Cognitive Enhancement 2, 388–396.

Laws, K. R. / Sweetnam, H. / Kondel, T. K. (2012): Is Ginkgo biloba a cognitive enhancer in healthy individuals? A meta-analysis. In: Human Psychopharmacology 27 (6), 527–533.

Lees, J. / Michalopoulou, P. G. / Lewis, S. W. / Preston, S. / Bamford, C. / Collier, T. / Kalpakidou, A. / Wykes, T. / Emsley, R. / Pandina, G. / Kapur, S. / Drake, R. J. (2017): Modafinil and cognitive enhancement in schizophrenia and healthy volunteers: the effects of test battery in a randomised controlled trial. In: Psychological Medicine 47 (13), 2358–2368.

Linssen, A. M. W. / Sambeth, A. / Vuurman, E. F. P. M. / Riedel, W. J. (2014): Cognitive effects of methylphenidate in healthy volunteers: a review of single dose studies. In: International Journal of Neuropsychopharmacology 17 (6), 961–977.

Lowe, C. J. / Safati, A. / Hall, P. A. (2017): The neurocognitive consequences of sleep restriction: A meta-analytic review. In: Neuroscience and Biobehavioral Reviews 80, 586–604.

Maher, B. (2008): Poll results: look who's doping. In: Nature 452 (7188), 674–675.

McKinley, R. A. / Bridges, N. / Walters, C. M. / Nelson, J. (2012): Modulating the brain at work using noninvasive transcranial stimulation. In: NeuroImage 59, 129–137.

Melby-Lervåg, M. / Redick, T. S. / Hulme C. (2016): Working memory training does not improve performance on measures of intelligence or other measures of »far transfer«: Evidence from a meta-analytic review. In: Perspectives on Psychological Science, 11 (4), 512–534.

Müller, G. / Freude, G. / Kersten, N. (2019): Neuroenhancement in Deutschland am Beispiel von vier Berufsgruppen. Neuroenhancement in four occupations in Germany. In: Gesundheitswesen, doi: 10.1055/a-1026-6157.

Nehlig, A. (2010): Is caffeine a cognitive enhancer? In: Journal of Alzheimer's Disease 20, 85–94.

Parkin, B. L. / Bhandari, M. / Glen, J. C. / Walsh, V. (2018): The physiological effects of transcranial electrical stimulation do not apply to parameters commonly used in studies of cognitive neuromodulation. In: Neuropsychologia 128, 332–339.

Polito, V. / Stevenson, R. J. (2019): A systematic study of microdosing psychedelics. In: PLoS ONE 14 (2), e0211023.

Prochazkova, L. / Lippelt, D. P. / Colzato, L. S. / Kuchar, M. / Sjoerds, Z. / Hommel, B. (2018) Exploring the effect of microdosing psychedelics on creativity in an open-label natural setting. In: Psychopharmacology 235, 3401–3413.

Repantis, D. / Laisney, O. / Heuser, I. (2010): Acetylcholinesterase inhibitors and memantine for neuroenhancement in healthy individuals: a systematic review. In: Pharmacological Research 61 (6), 473–481.

Roig, M. / Nordbrandt, S. / Geertsen, S. S. / Nielsen, J. B. (2013): The effects of cardiovascular exercise on human memory: a review with meta-analysis. In: Neuroscience & Biobehavioral Reviews 37 (8), 1645–1666.

Schilling, R. / Hoebel, J. / Müters, S. / Lange, C. (2012): Pharmakologisches Neuroenhancement. In: GBE kompakt 3 (3), ed. by Robert Koch-Institut Berlin.

Science Media Center Germany (ed.) (2019): Nicht-invasive Hirnstimulation – neue Möglichkeiten in Therapie und Forschung? Fact sheet. URL https://www.sciencemediacenter.de/alle-angebote/fact-sheet/details/news/nicht-invasive-hirnstimulation-neue-moeglichkeiten-in-therapie-und-forschung/ [25 November 2021].

Sedlmeier, P. / Eberth, J. / Schwarz, M. / Zimmermann, D. / Haarig, F. / Jaeger, S. / Kunze, S. (2012): The psychological effects of meditation: a meta-analysis. In: Psychological Bulletin 138 (6), 1139–1171.

Seinfeld, S. / Figueroa, H. / Ortiz-Gil, J. / Sanchez-Vives, M. V. (2013): Effects of music learning and piano practice on cognitive function, mood and quality of life in older adults. In: Frontiers in Psychology 4, 810.

Sellaro, R. / Derks, B. / Nitsche, M. A. / Hommel, B. / van den Wildenberg, W. P. M. / van Dam, K. / Colzato, L. S. (2015): Reducing Prejudice Through Brain Stimulation. In: Brain Stimulation 8 (5), 891–897.

Simons, D. J. / Boot, W. R. / Charness, N. / Gathercole, S. E. / Chabris, C. F. / Hambrick, D. Z. / Stine-Morrow, E. A. (2016): Do »brain-training« programs work? In: Psychological Science in the Public Interest 17 (3), 103–186.

Smillie, L. D. / Gökçen, E. (2010): Caffeine enhances working memory for extraverts. In: Biological Psychology 85 (3), 496–498.

Smith, P. J. / Blumenthal, J. A. / Hoffman, B. M. / Cooper, H. / Strauman, T. A. / Welsh-Bohmer, K. / Browndyke, J. N. / Sherwood, A. (2010): Aerobic Exercise and Neurocognitive Performance: A Meta-Analytic Review of Randomized Controlled Trials. In: Psychosomatic Medicine 72 (3), 239–252.

Smith, M. A. / Riby, L. M. / Eekelen, J. A. / Foster, J. K. (2011): Glucose enhancement of human memory: a comprehensive research review of the glucose memory facilitation effect. In: Neuroscience & Biobehavioral Reviews 35 (3), 770–783.

Stojanoski, B. / Lyons, K. M. / Pearce, A. A. A. / Owen, A. M. (2018): Targeted training: Converging evidence against the transferable benefits of online brain training on cognitive function. In: Neuropsychologia 117, 541–550.

Suthana, N. / Haneef, Z. / Stern, J. / Mukamel, R. / Behnke, E. / Knowlton, B. / Fried, I. (2012): Memory Enhancement and Deep-Brain Stimulation of the Entorhinal Area. In: The New England Journal of Medicine 366, 502–510.

Tardif, S. / Simard, M. (2011): Cognitive Stimulation Programs in Healthy Elderly: A Review. In: International Journal of Alzheimer's Disease, 378934.

Thibaut, A. / Zafonte, R. / Morse, L. R. / Fregni, F. (2017): Understanding Negative Results in tDCS Research: The Importance of Neural Targeting and Cortical Engagement. In: Frontiers in Neuroscience 11, 707.

Tildesley, N. T. / Kennedy, D. O. / Perry, E. K. / Ballard, C. G. / Savelev, S. / Wesnes, K. A. / Scholey, A. B. (2003): Salvia lavandulaefolia (Spanish sage) enhances memory in healthy young volunteers. In: Pharmacology Biochemistry and Behavior 75 (3), 669–674.

Valentine, G. / Sofuoglu, M. (2018): Cognitive Effects of Nicotine: Recent Progress. In: Current Neuropharmacology 16 (4), 403–414.

Warburton, D. M. (1992): Nicotine as a cognitive enhancer. In: Progress in Neuro-Psychopharmacology and Biological Psychiatry 16 (2), 181–191.

Warwick, K. (2014): The Cyborg Revolution. In: NanoEthics 8, 263–273.

Yanakieva, S. / Polychroni, N. / Family, N. / Williams, L. T. J. / Luke, D. P. / Terhune, D. B. (2019): The effects of microdose LSD on time perception: a randomised, double-blind, placebo-controlled trial. In: Psychopharmacology 236, 1159–1170.

Yetisen, A. K. (2018): Biohacking. In: Trends in Biotechnology 36 (8), 744–747.

II. Ethics of Neuroenhancement

Jan-Hendrik Heinrichs, Markus Rüther, Mandy Stake

1.___Introduction

Human enhancement is one of the most controversially debated topics in current bioethics. The contemporary debate started in the late 1990s and has yet to show signs of abating.[1] Time and again, developments in science and engineering have been the catalyst for ethical contributions. Cosmetic surgery[2] and administration of a synthetic human growth hormone[3] have been among the first technologies to set hopes and concerns with human enhancement. Shortly after, genetic manipulation became the focus of attention in the debate[4], only to be outflanked by neuroenhancement, i.e. means that are designed to improve mental capacities such as neuro-pharmaceuticals and neuro-technologies.[5]

In the following, our aim is to give an overview of this last trend in the enhancement debate. Due to the extensive literature and different perspectives on the subject, it is by no means a straightforward task. Therefore, it seems to be necessary to mention at least a few caveats in order to make our presuppositions and restrictions transparent.

First, it is important to notice that the debate about human enhancement in general and neuroenhancement in particular has not just been an ethical and philosophical, but also a political endeavour from the beginning onward. Several of the major contributions are either explicitly intended as policy advice[6] or take recourse to a legalistic conception of what ethics does.[7] Their ethical arguments aim at legal regulation, e.g. suggesting that the use of technologies, which can support certain forms of moral motivation or deliberation, should be made obligatory for future genera-

---

[1] Erik Parens narrates the start of the modern debate in the introduction of Parens 1998b.
[2] Cf. Little 1998.
[3] Cf. Haverkamp / Ranke 1999.
[4] Cf. Silver 1997; Harris 1992.
[5] Cf. Farah et al. 2004.
[6] Cf. e.g. Parens 1998b; President's Council on Bioethics (U.S.) 2003.
[7] Cf. Friele 2008.

tions.[8] Given the strong policy suggestions formulated by several authors, it is of little surprise that participants in this debate have been sorted into camps, labelled with terms originating in politics, mostly US politics. It has become common fare to refer to the main contributors to the debate as bio-conservatives, bio-liberals, bio-moderates and transhumanists. These labels, however, have repeatedly called into question for good reasons.[9] In previous publications we decided to refer to permissive, restrictive and mandatory positions and will stick to this distinction here.[10]

Secondly, many contributions to the enhancement debate took their start with policy suggestions for particular technologies or uses, e. g. enhancement via *genetic editing*, or *moral* enhancement. They attended to what the authors took as the advent of a specific new technology and the replies as well as the consecutive debates focused on this particular technology and its application. When for example recombinant production of the human growth hormone became possible and first results suggested it might be efficient in combating non-pathological low body height and might even have anti-aging effects[11], it became the topic of a fairly specific debate which included detailed regulatory suggestions. When it turned out that Prozac—and similar drugs—improved the mood of people without depressive disorder, it became the topic of a large body of literature, which suggested ways of regulating and using antidepressants, but which often did not draw conclusions for other types of enhancement.[12] Many overviews of the enhancement debate follow the individual strands of discussions about individual enhancement projects and are structured accordingly. For example, one of the more comprehensive editions on human enhancement is structured into the sections »cognitive enhancement«, »mood enhancement«, »physical enhancement«, »lifespan extension« and »moral enhancement«.[13] While this is a natural approach to the topic, it tends to introduce a certain redundancy in the arguments presented. Many arguments on the ethical standing of human enhancement have been applied or are applicable to different forms of enhancement. We will follow a different path here and structure our discussion of the state of the debate along the different supporting or counterarguments which have been brought forth.

---

[8] Cf. Persson / Savulescu 2008.

[9] Cf. e. g. Parens 2005: 35; Macklin 2006. Other terminological suggestions such as Caplan's ›meliorists‹ and ›anti-meliorists‹ have not really caught on, cf. Caplan 2009.

[10] Cf. Heinrichs / Stake 2018; Rüther / Heinrichs 2019; Heinrichs / Stake 2019.

[11] Cf. Rudman et al. 1990.

[12] Cf. Kramer 1994.

[13] Savulescu / ter Meulen / Kahane 2011.

Thirdly, the various strands of highly specific arguments have been the nucleus of the modern enhancement debate, but they obviously do not exhaust the contributions to the topic. More general contributions soon started to enrich the debate. Authors did not merely focus on specific technologies and their uses, but identified a general trend and interrelated moral issues, which have been discussed under the general term ›enhancement‹. For instance, authors analysed reasons for or against enhancement as an individual life choice. In particular, debates about the authenticity of using enhancement and about specific enhancement's effects on the user's character targeted the individual pursuit of a good life beyond any social or political impact. Furthermore, authors tried to support moral deliberation in private interaction by providing reasons to blame or praise others—and oneself—for engaging in enhancement without even claiming that these reasons were suitable for the design of sanction-reinforced rules. Due to this trend, we adjust our perspective on the debate. Thus, we try to successively and systematically broaden the perspective of our overview by introducing a differentiation that separates the objects of the different arguments in the realms of the individual's good life, his social interaction and—of course—the locus classicus of policy advice.

Methodologically, we explore the topic in the following way: we start out with some preliminary and mostly technical sections on the targets (sec. 2) and means (sec. 3) of enhancement, also highlighting the struggle in finding an appropriate definition of enhancement (sec. 4). This will serve as a solid background for the ethical discussion which will be the main part of this volume (sec. 5). In this part, we aim at giving an elaborate and in-depth analysis of the current state of the art. Last but not least, we conclude our overview with a short summary which is followed by a few thoughts on the shortcomings and future »work package« for participants of the debate (sec. 6).

2.___What can be enhanced?
On the targets of (neuro-)enhancement

Enhancement has its roots in a patchwork of fairly specific projects of improving specific bodily, cognitive and emotive functions together with the above-mentioned moral debates about these projects. The general technical term ›enhancement‹ has emerged rather recently, most of these specific projects have been pursued long before there was a coherent enhancement-debate, much less a definition of enhancement[14] and its sub-categories of neuroenhancement, doping, or genetic enhancement etc.

The number of human body functions which have meanwhile been targeted with the aim of being enhanced is immense. Most prominently, the age-old dream of extending the human life-span has not only manifested in mythical motives like the philosopher's stone or the fountain of youth, which is already mentioned by Herodotus in *The Histories*, Book 3.[15] It has also driven medical research from antiquity until today. As anti-aging technologies typically do not fall under the scope of neuroenhancement, we will not discuss them in much detail here. It should, however, be mentioned that several neuroenhancement technologies will most likely be part of the package of anti-aging technologies, insofar as they can counter mental effects of aging.[16] The dream of extending the healthy lifespan has been accompanied for an equally long time by the hope to gain greater bodily strength, dexterity and fortitude. The latest state of the art is not exactly easy to identify, because in recent years there has been a race between anti-doping agencies and agents in favour of doping who create means and methods of improving athletic performance which are either not yet banned or cannot be detected. However, a good overview of the recent state of the art is readily accessible in the continuously updated list of doping methods provided by the World Anti-Doping Association (WADA) on their website.[17]

The only comparison the previous two aims need to fear is that to the search for enhancing sexual pleasures. Even before the advent of modern Viagra, sexual enhancement has been continuously pursued since ancient times, e.g. by the use of drugs or foods.[18] However, these traditional targets of real and fictional enhancement-interventions have been overshadowed by the improvement of cognitive functions and mood enhancement in recent decades. The latter are often subsumed under the heading of ›neuroenhancement‹, but have for the most part been around well before this term was coined. The term seems to start to occur in scientific publishing in 2004.[19] The targets of neuroenhancement can roughly be categorized into cognition and mood. Two additional mixed categories

---

[14] Cf. section 4 (»What is enhancement? On the definition of enhancement«).

[15] Herodotus 2013.

[16] A detailed discussion of the philosophical dimensions of anti-aging technologies can be found in: Knell 2015.

[17] WADA 2020.

[18] Cf. Cosman 1983.

[19] Cf. Schleim / Quednow 2018: figure 1.

—moral and love enhancement—are sometimes added to the primary targets.

Cognition

Common targets of the enhancement of cognitive functions are perception, attention including concentration, understanding, memory, reasoning including creativity, and coordination of motor output. More specific cognitive functions are mentioned in some articles, as for example »the capacity to understand and appreciate music, humour, eroticism, narration, spirituality, mathematics, etc.«.[20] The field of cognitive enhancement has become so wide that it merits its own academic journal, the *Journal of Cognitive Enhancement*, which treats such diverse means as physical exercise, meditation, genetic editing, electromagnetic stimulation as well as psychopharmaceuticals and their effects on different cognitive processes. In real world practice, the most common version of cognitive enhancement seems to be psychopharmaceuticals targeted at improving attention span and wakefulness.[21]

Mood

While there has always been extensive effort to improve mood by chemical means, few of these attempts have received much attention beyond the literature on drug abuse for a long time. More recently, however, the modification of mood via antidepressants and other medical means has been greeted with interest by the general audience. Mood enhancement has not yet been differentiated into subtypes with the same efforts as attempts to improve cognition. Typically, authors discussing mood enhancement focus on the three main practical examples, i.e. mood improvements via antidepressants[22], reduction of anxiety either by anxiolytics or via heart medication, especially beta-blockers[23], and promoting trust and pro-social attitudes by oxytocin.[24] There are suggestions that inducing negative moods might be a form of mood enhancement as well, if it serves to fit a person's mood to her circumstances, such as allowing someone to grieve.[25]

---

[20] Bostrom 2008: 108.
[21] Cf. Maier / Ferris / Winstock 2018.
[22] Cf. Kramer 1994.
[23] Cf. Kahane 2011.
[24] Cf. Douglas 2008.
[25] Cf. Kahane 2011.

Morality
Another large category of biotechnological interventions that find ample attention under the heading of neuroenhancement is moral enhancement, where the use of drugs is discussed to either modify motives for moral behaviour in the widest sense, or to enable moral insight. It is not always clear how moral enhancement is to be kept apart from cognitive and mood enhancement, because it aims to modify states of the human mind which play a specific role in moral situations, but typically are not moral *per se*.[26] Thus, characterising an enhancement as ›moral‹ tries to cluster the interventions according to their role in a complex social practice and not according to some schema used in the cognitive sciences as the categories ›cognitive‹ and ›mood‹ do.[27]

Love
The same holds true for the last subcategory of neuroenhancement, the so-called *love enhancement*[28] which seems to combine forms of cognitive, moral, and emotional enhancement and would be applied to couples rather than to individuals under the right circumstances.

Much as ›moral enhancement‹, this taxonomic suggestion seems to cluster together very different interventions. We therefore suggest sticking to the differentiation between cognitive and mood enhancement for taxonomic reasons, while admitting that some types of enhancement will result in changes which are morally relevant or have an effect on the love life of human beings.

3.____How to enhance? On the means of enhancement

The patchwork of individual enhancement projects that finally sparked the general enhancement debate was not merely scattered across different functions, but also across different means of enhancement. In many cases the advent of biotechnological means for aims that had already been pursued by other means generated attention and ethical scrutiny. Take for example growth: parents have tried to induce growth in their children

---

[26] Cf. Beck 2015; Douglas 2008; Persson / Savulescu 2008.
[27] Given the complexity of morality, the authors take it to be questionable whether employing the term ›moral‹ as a sorting scheme for enhancement interventions has any taxonomic advantage at all. The same holds for the term ›love enhancement‹. Again, the phenomenon in question is too broad to generate a useful taxonomic category, unless one reduces the phenomenon to a very limited set of its components.
[28] Savulescu / Sandberg 2008: 38.

for quite some time. They used such whimsical methods as having them stand in summer rain, or common sense measures such as physical activity and decent nutrition, going into details such as suggesting to practice yoga and drink extra portions of milk. None of these methods ever made it into an article in a philosophical journal, but the use of growth hormone immediately did.[29] And it raised awareness for the detrimental effects of body ideals, which nobody ever talked about when everything we had were nutrition, exercise, and summer rain. The same effect can be observed for other technologies and products: nobody cared for kids taking pure dextrose into exams, but Ritalin made it into lead articles of philosophical journals; coffee gets sold in unlimited doses in many schools as well as all universities and nobody even notices, but Modafinil has been discussed widely in scholarly articles, etc.

What grew into the enhancement debate has originally revolved around specific biotechnological interventions, nearly all of which have originally been introduced for therapeutic, preventive of palliative purposes. Reference to enhancement as an encompassing concept and even to so-called *enhancement technologies* settled in when commonalities of different individual improvement projects were identified. Accordingly, it should be kept in mind that there is no such thing as an enhancement technology. Each of the technologies involved can be used for different purposes such as therapy, torture, palliation, poisoning, or enhancement. Thus, loose talk about enhancement technologies is (or should be) intended to refer to technologies which can be or are used for enhancement purposes and to the marketing of biomedical technologies for enhancement purposes.

Unsurprisingly, most biomedical technologies which can be used for enhancement purposes have been used this way. In the following, we will focus on the ethical debates about neurotechnologies, i.e. technologies affecting the nervous system, thus neglecting other technologies, which are extensively used for aesthetic and sports enhancement, such as surgery and blood doping. However, many of the arguments which concern neuroenhancement are also applicable and have indeed been applied to other forms of enhancement, even if the overlap is not perfect.

The technologies that have sparked most ethical debates about neuroenhancement fall into three large categories, namely psychopharmaceuticals, neurostimulation, and genetic manipulation. Each of these categories encompasses a plethora of individual technologies and substances

---

[29] For a history of enhancement with human growth hormone in sports, cf. Holt et al. 2009. For its use in paediatric enhancement, cf. Morrison 2015.

as well as their applications, which we cannot discuss in any detail here. The most commonly used class of neuroenhancement is psychopharmaceuticals. While some authors insist that only legal drugs used for non-therapeutic purposes should be considered as enhancement, we want to widen this scope to other substances. Neither their legality nor registration as a drug, which depend on national context anyway[30], seem to make a significant difference to a substance's suitability for enhancement use. Illegal substances such as LSD or psilocybin are used for enhancement purposes, as are substances such as caffeine, which most cultures consider a food item and not a drug.[31]

The enhancement debate has reached a point where it does not exclusively focus on the technologies which have in fact been used for enhancement purposes. Rather, there is ample discussion—often speculative—about possible uses of established therapeutic technologies for enhancement and about the use of merely possible technologies, such as drugs, without adverse effects. A good example of the former is the debate about the enhancement use of invasive brain stimulation technologies, in particular about Deep Brain Stimulation (DBS). For obvious reasons intracranial stimulation technologies, i.e. technologies which are implanted within the cranium, are not suited for home use or casual enhancement projects. They require surgery together with the whole infrastructure that goes with it. The high risk associated with these invasive technologies is not easily compensated for by potential benefits of enhancement. The enhancing effect would have to be very large for this. At the moment, the risks associated with invasive neurostimulation are balanced by therapeutic effects in otherwise untreatable serious diseases such as Parkinson's disease or epilepsy. Nevertheless, there has been extensive discussion about possible enhancement use of DBS.[32] Similarly cognitive enhancement via genetic editing is not a contemporary technological option[33], which does not hinder some of the most prominent authors discussing their potential for such use.[34]

---

[30] Cf. e.g. King 2013.
[31] An impressive overview of the enhancing effects of diverse legal and illegal substances can be found in Müller / Schumann 2011. Nevertheless, legality is an important moral issue: While it can and should be debated whether certain substances should be illegal, the fact that they are illegal should be a moral reason not to produce, obtain, distribute, or use them.
[32] Cf. e.g. Synofzik / Schlaepfer 2008.
[33] For an overview cf. Lavazza 2018b.
[34] Cf. Buchanan 2011b; Harris 2007.

4.___What is enhancement? On the definition of enhancement

If indeed ethical arguments on enhancement have repeatedly been provoked by relevant new technologies, we should think that we have quite
a clear concept of enhancement. However, it turned out in detailed discussions that this is not the case. What is meant by ›enhancement‹ and which
technologies fall under the term has been hotly contested for years and
there is still no clear consensus on this issue. Positions on this question
are disparate enough that even the famous solution of Potter Stewart »I
know it when I see it«[35] does not work. Different authors referring to the
same physical objects or procedures come to very different conclusions as
to whether they can be categorized as enhancement.

The reason for these differences in categorization is simple: ›enhancement‹ is not a term to describe natural kinds, but a term used to contrast
certain uses of techniques and technologies from others for quite different
purposes.[36] In medical practice, the term ›enhancement‹ is being used to
contrast successful interventions from unsuccessful ones, that is, it refers
to any biotechnological intervention that brings about improvement in
some physiological or psychological function. Outside the field of medicine, ›enhancement‹ has been introduced to refer to forms of non-stan-
dard uses of medical means as opposed to their standard use in prevention, diagnosis, therapy, and palliation.[37] Depending on their stance on
the use of biomedical technologies beyond these standard uses of medicine, some authors label enhancement as a misuse or abuse of medical
technologies. This difference between therapy and enhancement lingers
in most attempts at a definition.

As mentioned, the definition of enhancement has been approached
from significantly different angles, which can be grouped into four different strands which we will discuss respectively: 1) the ›beyond therapy‹-
strand, 2) the ›beyond species-typical functioning‹-strand, 3) the ›welfarist‹-strand, and 4) the ›umbrella-term‹-strand.[38]

---

[35] Cf. Lattman 2007.
[36] Cf. Heinrichs 2017.
[37] Cf. Parens 1998a.
[38] Cf. Savulescu / ter Meulen / Kahane 2011.

4.1 ›Beyond therapy‹-strand

The beyond therapy strand contrasts the use of medical technologies for enhancement against that for therapy.[39] This strand has been dominant in early approaches to enhancement, especially in the notorious report by the US President's Council on Bioethics *Beyond therapy*. It starts its fairly detailed discussion of what enhancement is with the following rough definition:

»›Therapy,‹ on this view as in common understanding, is the use of biotechnical power to treat individuals with known diseases, disabilities, or impairments, in an attempt to restore them to a normal state of health and fitness. ›Enhancement,‹ by contrast, is the directed use of biotechnical power to alter, by direct intervention, not disease processes but the ›normal‹ workings of the human body and psyche, to augment or improve their native capacities and performances.«[40]

It has been quickly pointed out that a reference to health for distinguishing between therapy and what goes beyond it presupposes a clear distinction between healthy and non-healthy states. Such a distinction is typically provided by a theory of health, a topic in the philosophy of medicine which is still debated.[41] However, the ›beyond therapy‹-strand does not need to turn on the distinction between health and disease. It is possible to give an account of the terms ›treatment‹ and ›therapy‹ without reference to ›health‹ or ›disease‹, or to take ›therapy‹ as a primary term within this context which does not need any further explication. The conceptual origin of ›therapy‹ in the ancient Greek ›therapeía‹ refers first of all to service and care. These can be provided for quite different reasons than the illness of the person being cared for. The conceptual origin of ›treat‹ in Latin ›trahere‹ refers to forms of bodily care, in particular to the provision with food. The medical use actually seems to have developed later. If one takes these origins seriously, then the therapy or treatment of disease would only be a sub-form of the care of bodily needs or care. In both cases, ›therapy‹ can be used as a contrast term to ›enhancement‹ without opening up debates about the concept ›health‹.

---

[39] Cf. e. g. Juengst 1998.
[40] President's Council on Bioethics (U.S.) 2003: 13.
[41] Cf. e. g. Schramme 2017.

4.2 ›Beyond species-typical functioning‹-strand

The second strand, the ›beyond species-typical functioning‹-strand, defines uses of a given technology as enhancement if they enable functioning beyond what is typical for the species. Uses of the same technology is not considered enhancement but therapy if they enable functioning up to what is typical for the species.[42]

To put it more precisely, according to this strand, enhancement by biotechnological means is enabling human beings to function on a level beyond what is considered as normal for their comparison group. This definition strongly depends on a clarification of the functions it refers to and the conception of normality it uses. As both ›function‹ and ›normality‹ are contested terms in the philosophy of biology, philosophy of mind, and in ethics, a plethora of slightly divergent concepts is available. ›Function‹ has been limited to core biological functions of reproduction and survival[43], extended to broader biological functions including psychological functions[44] and interpreted broadly in order to include diverse cognitive, artistic, social and other functions. ›Normality‹ has been interpreted in a strong theoretical sense[45] as well as in a purely statistical sense.[46]

The ›beyond‹ in ›beyond species-typical functioning‹ is being alluded to in the name for the single most homogeneous group of authors that actively promotes human enhancement: transhumanists. The ›trans‹ in ›transhumanism‹ refers— amongst others—to going above the functions human beings can normally realise. This term catches the idea of the ›beyond species-average‹ strand quite accurately, if sometimes slightly exaggerated:

»You have just celebrated your 170th birthday and you feel stronger than ever. Each day is a joy. You have invented entirely new art forms, which exploit the new kinds of cognitive capacities and sensibilities you have developed. You still listen to music—music that is to Mozart what Mozart is to bad Muzak. You are communicating with your contemporaries using a language that has grown out of English over the past century and that has a vocabulary and expressive power that enables you to share and discuss thoughts and feelings that unaugmented humans could not even think or experience.«[47]

---

[42] Cf. e.g. Daniels / Sabin 1997.
[43] Cf. Boorse 1977.
[44] Cf. Boorse 1976.
[45] Cf. Daniels / Sabin 1997.
[46] Cf. Boorse 1977.
[47] Bostrom 2008: 112.

There is a close theoretical relation between the first two strands of definition. This relation owes to the fact that species typical functioning is one of the core definitions of health in the philosophy of medicine.[48] To be precise, the two definitional strands refer to the same contrast if 1) therapy is understood as combating or alleviating diseases or disorders, and 2) disease and disorder are defined with regard to species-typical functioning. The contrast in question is between improvement up to the species-typical level (therapy) vs. improvement beyond species-typical functioning (enhancement). This relation is contingent. One can insist that enhancement is any use of biomedical technology beyond therapy without any reference to species-typical function. Vice versa, it is possible to define enhancement as biotechnologically enabling functioning beyond species-typical levels and not refer back to a concept of therapy at all.

4.3 Welfarism

The ›welfarist‹-strand of definitions neither makes use of the concept of therapy nor of species-typical functioning. It defines enhancement as biological or psychological changes in a person that increase her welfare, i. e. her probability of leading a good life.[49] The terms ›welfare‹ and ›good life‹ need some explication. Authors who use the welfarist definition have taken recourse to hedonistic, to desire-fulfilment, and even to evolutionary fitness-based theories for that. Given that the formulation above would include breakfast and hearing a good joke, most authors limit enhancement to biological or psychological changes brought about by the use of biotechnological means.[50]

Unlike the previous definitions, the ›welfarist‹-strand is not suited to draw a distinction between therapy and enhancement. Therapies will have to be considered as one type of enhancement, which only gradually differs from other improvements of human well-being by biotechnological means. Again, unlike the previous definitions, the ›welfarist‹-strand has a close affinity to an ethical position. The welfarist definition is typically used in context of utilitarian evaluations of biotechnologies. In this context, the use of the welfarist definition runs the risk of prejudicing the results: while the moral value of enhancements can be topped by arguments from distributive justice, adverse side effects or similar secondary

---

[48] Cf. Boorse 1977.
[49] Cf. e. g. Savulescu / Sandberg / Kahane 2011.
[50] Cf. Heilinger 2010.

effects, it cannot turn out to be negative itself. This has been pointed out by John Harris, who insists that »If it wasn't good for you, it wouldn't be enhancement.«[51]

4.4 Umbrella term

The last definitional strand has been called »sociological pragmatic«[52] or an »umbrella term«-concept.[53] The core idea of this definitional strand is that what falls under ›enhancement‹ is decided by common practices of valuing, financing, and using medical technologies. At least in common usage, neither ›therapy‹ nor ›enhancement‹ is a term with a homogeneous reference. What is accepted as a proper part of standard medical therapy is not explained by any of the approaches above, but rather by what counts as normal within a given society. People consider interventions as standard medical care which are not preventive, diagnostic, therapeutic, or palliative, and they exclude some uses which clearly are. This heterogeneous practice of applying biomedical technologies for quite diverse goals has been taken up with the term ›compensatory enhancement‹, which is intended to refer to uses of biomedical techniques that re-establish normal functioning without being strictly therapeutic.[54]

Following this strand, the reference of ›enhancement‹ is not given by some definite description or even a definition, but by its use in a broad set of contexts. This sounds like a surprising turn not just in content but in method as well. Unlike all the previous strands, understanding ›enhancement‹ as umbrella term goes along with different semantic implications: in contrast to terms depicting natural kinds with a closely circumscribed reference or a theoretical term that is introduced by an explicit definition, umbrella terms obtain their meaning from their actual usage in language. Thus, the meaning of ›enhancement‹ understood as umbrella term being under consideration particularly in the fields of ethics, biotechnology, and medicine, is constituted by the different forms of usage in these contexts. However, while this approach might be the most accurate regarding its underlying theory of meaning as well as regarding the meaning of ›enhancement‹, it does not even attempt to establish a unified definition or allow for more general claims about enhancement.

---

51 Harris 2007: 9.
52 Savulescu / Sandberg / Kahane 2011: 3 f.
53 Chadwick 2009: 30 f.
54 Cf. Birnbacher 2012: 113 f.

4.5 Commonalities

A common denominator of the competing enhancement definitions is their reference to biotechnological interventions. Only biotechnological interventions are considered as enhancements, not everything that is ›good for you‹ (John Harris) or ›enhances human traits‹ (Erik Parens): Neither a decent breakfast[55] nor a lesson in mnemonics is considered a kind of enhancement, if most authors in the debate are to be followed.[56] It has, however, been suggested that some external devices are at least analogous to enhancement. Harris considers the case of glasses and Nick Bostrom and Anders Sandberg discuss computing and information technology.[57] But neither Harris nor Bostrom and Sandberg make use of their broader understanding of enhancement when discussing the ethics of enhancement. The relevant sections refer to the ethics of biotechnological enhancement only. Bostrom and Sandberg's finer categorization into types of enhancement reveals the exceptional status of external devices: they distinguish conventional means of enhancement such as education and training from unconventional means, namely »nootropic drugs, gene therapy, or neural implants«.[58] External devices are neither here nor there, conventional means are widely ignored in the ethical argumentation. There often are good reasons for this focus, such as the mere novelty of biotechnological means and the resulting moral uncertainty of how to deal with them. But as Allen Buchanan pointed out, focusing on biomedical technologies alone runs a certain risk of biomedical exceptionalism for which there seem to be no adequate reasons.[59]

5. Ethical Arguments – for and against

We will present the arguments in a specific order by differentiating between arguments which are concerned with the individual on her own (5.1), her dialogical interaction with others (5.2), and arguments which focus on the society as a whole and appropriate policy advice (5.3). How-

---

[55] Cf. Heilinger 2010.

[56] Allen Buchanan is one prominent author, who counts any action as enhancement »that improves some capacity (or characteristic) that normal human beings ordinarily have or, more radically, that produces a new one« (Buchanan 2011a: 5). He then quickly distinguishes between biomedical and other forms of enhancement.

[57] Cf. Bostrom / Sandberg 2009.

[58] Ibid.: 312.

[59] Cf. Buchanan 2011a: 5.

ever, note that the order in which we will present the arguments owes to internal interdependencies. Many arguments which are presented as policy advice owe their argumentative force to the fact that they identify reasons which a person might take into account in her individual deliberation about the pursuit of a good life, if she were fully informed and deliberated with great care. Take for example the suggestion to ban certain substances from enhancement use because of their adverse effects. If this suggestion refers to the person harming herself—as opposed to harming others by production and distribution—then it owes all its plausibility to the fact that persons might, given a common preference set, have reason to avoid this harm. If people did not have reason to avoid such harm, there would be no ground for the policy suggestion in question.

This direction of interdependence is fairly common within the debate, which is why we will start our presentation with reasons for and against enhancement which play a role in individual deliberation about the pursuit of a good life. Only then will we broaden the scope of affected parties, go into reasons for deliberation about social conduct and private interaction and finally discuss reasons for social policy.

5.1   *Enhancement and the individual good life*

The debate about human enhancement is one of the bioethical domains in which the individual good life has played a dominant role from early on. In other debates of bioethics, there is a stronger emphasis on questions of self-determination and autonomy or on welfare as understood in therapeutic endeavours.[60] The latter concepts, in turn, tend to play a minor role in the enhancement debate, in particular because the standard cases of enhancement affects competent adults whose decision-making capacity is not compromised by any medical condition. As a consequence, there is a more detailed discussion about the contribution of biotechnological interventions to an individual's good life than in many other areas of bioethics. This has additional novelty value insofar as many of the biotechnological interventions discussed under the label of enhancement are highly regulated under medical or drug law. The suggestion that they might have benefits for healthy individuals has—especially for the substances regulated under drug legislation—been constrained to mostly non-academic debates about drug legalisation.[61]

---

[60] Cf. Kipke 2013.
[61] Cf. Heinrichs / Stake 2018.

5.1.1 Supporting arguments

5.1.1.1 *Improved welfare*

Nobody would have felt the necessity to debate the moral standing of enhancement if it did not hold the promise of individual welfare gains. An increasingly large number of people has come to perceive biotechnologies as suitable tools for improving their daily lives beyond their medical needs. This trend has been caught up by authors in philosophy, who systematised the different possible benefits of such enhancement use. In some cases, this systematising effort went hand in hand with strongly favourable evaluations of enhancement use of biomedical technologies, in other cases such individual benefits have been drawn into doubt and characterised as either spurious[62], morally corrupt[63], or outweighed by possible harm.[64]

Identifying the individual benefits of biotechnological enhancements is the core strategy of any consequentialist argument concerning these interventions. This is why the counterclaim, namely that there are no such benefits, has been met with incredulity. Several authors have expressed their irritation at the fact that biotechnological enhancement is not accepted as clearly beneficial for the user. Harris wonders:

»Our question is this: if the goal of enhanced intelligence, increased powers and capacities, and better health is something that we might strive to produce through education, including of course the more general health education of the community, why should we not produce these goals, if we can do so safely, through enhancement technologies or procedures?«[65]

Allen Buchanan raises the same point:

»*Biomedical* enhancements have provoked huge controversy. Given that enhancement isn't new and that it has played a central role in human progress, what's all the fuss? Why should we tie our hands, cut ourselves off from further progress, by forgoing enhancements just because they happen to use biomedical technologies?«[66]

Similarly, in Germany Dieter Birnbacher asked:

»Why then, one will have to ask, the particular controversy of enhancement? Is it not part of technology as such that it transforms and transforms that which exists ›by nature‹ according to human needs, even without there being a ›necessity‹, an

---

[62] Cf. Elliott 1998.
[63] Cf. Sandel 2007.
[64] Cf. Chatterjee 2004.
[65] Harris 2007: 2.
[66] Buchanan 2011a: 12.

immediately compelling need for it? What is questionable about the fact that the means of biomedicine are also used for this purpose? Does it not seem surprising that in the majority of public debates on enhancement, the burden of proof is not placed on those who wish to restrict the freedom to enhance, but on those who defend this freedom?«[67]

These authors are open for a *pro tanto* negative verdict about biotechnological enhancement. It might turn out that the advantages get overcompensated by disadvantages, but they insist that there are still obvious advantages which merit close attention.

Following Buchanan, the promises of biotechnological enhancement can be distinguished into two types of benefit[68]: intrinsic benefits of cognitive enhancement, referring to the fact that activities and states enabled by cognitive enhancements are valued for their own sake, and instrumental benefits of cognitive enhancement, meaning that cognitively enhanced persons will be able to generate more social value than the unenhanced. We will address them in this order.

Several states and activities seem to be valued—according to authors in the debate who otherwise agree on very little—for their own sake, most prominently life and health, knowledge and cognition, as well as pleasure and aesthetic appreciation.[69] Exactly these states and activities have been identified by several authors as possible targets of biotechnological enhancement. The most well-known article in this regard is Bostrom's *Why I want to be a posthuman when I grow up*, a sweeping endorsement of enhancement.[70] Bostrom takes up the challenge of showing whether biotechnologically induced gains in these activities and states would be good for the individual.

For each of these states and processes (healthy life, cognition, emotion), Bostrom provides evidence that improvements would be valued by possible beneficiaries and in particular by those who we would consider good judges in the matter. Given that such improvements would be valued in general, Bostrom infers that the same is true for biotechnologically induced improvements. His examples for improvements start out with common hopes such as improved concentration span or better memory. He quickly moves on to more complex abilities such as improved transparency of the justification of one's own beliefs and he ends with fairly

---

[67] Birnbacher 2012: 112. Translation by Jan-Hendrik Heinrichs.

[68] Buchanan 2011b: 117 ff.

[69] Hauskeller and Sandel would accept the intrinsic value of most of these items just as Bostrom does. In the wider literature, these items regularly occur on so-called *objective lists of human welfare*, cf. Alkire 2002: 87 ff. for an overview.

[70] Cf. Bostrom 2008.

remote possibilities which seem to overstress the descriptive ability of even such an eloquent writer as Bostrom. He avoids clear descriptions by pointing to the limitation of the present powers of our imagination:

»If, aside from extended health spans, the essence of posthumanity is to be able to have thoughts and experiences that we cannot readily think or experience with our current capacities, then it is not surprising that our ability to imagine what post-human life might be like is very limited.«[71]

Bostrom makes a point of addressing authors who claim that the benefits of enhancement are spurious or generally outbalanced by its harms. Thus, while they might feel the same irritation expressed by Buchanan, Harris and Birnbacher try to explain and refute the reasons for disclaiming the benefits of enhancements. The five types of reasons Harris discusses are 1) the impossibility of implementation, 2) the cost of implementation, 3) negative impacts on society, 4) outbalancing harms, and 5) discontinuity or lack of identity. The first three of these reasons are not suited to show that enhancement does not generate benefits for its users, they merely show that these benefits—if the whole endeavour is feasible—will not come for free. The fourth reason is the core target of the article. As described above, Bostrom provides several pieces of evidence that the benefits brought about by biotechnological enhancement would be valued by actual persons. The fifth and last reason has been discussed at the outset of the debate but has been quickly refuted. The original idea was imported from the theory of personal identity, claiming that a person, who is unenhanced at one point in time, and the same person, who has undergone enhancement in the meanwhile, are not identical or not sufficiently psychologically continuous in order to say that the original person has gained anything by possible benefits in the life of the enhanced person. Bostrom refers to Walter Glannon[72] as one author suggesting such a theory.

Claims that enhancement might endanger personal identity such as that of Glannon have been scrutinized in some details by David DeGrazia. He argued as one of the first proponents of enhancement that »there's no reason to think enhancing an existing person's cognitive and affective abilities would affect numerical identity«[73] or »violate an untouchable core«[74]. He insists that identity endangering alterations of per-

---

[71] Bostrom 2008: 112.
[72] Cf. Glannon 2002.
[73] DeGrazia 2005: 267.
[74] Ibid.: 272.

50

sonal identity by enhancement methods need to be addressed within a framework of narrative identity. He rejects mere references to changes in biological structure as endangering identity, simply because human organisms change continuously anyway. Thus, one would have to argue that enhancement interventions can and are likely to affect so-called *core traits*, which he takes to be (i) internal personal style, (ii) intelligence, (iii) normal functioning, especially normal ageing, (iv) gender, and (v) being homo sapiens. DeGrazia quickly rejects claims (i) and (ii) by pointing out that »both genetic and environmental interventions affect the properties of our brain.«[75] He does not see why »manipulating the environment to improve intelligence is acceptable«, whereas »possibly more efficacious means to the same laudable end [are taken to] be problematic.«[76] In arguing against (iii) as a core trait he states that »even if aging [sic!] is an inviolable core trait of human beings, living no more than some specified number of years is not.«[77] While DeGrazia accepts—according to (iv)—that gender »may be crucial to someone's narrative identity at a particular time,« he also stresses that »gender is not critical to numerical identity.«[78] In response to (v), DeGrazia criticizes every step in the argument of restrictive views as mistaken since even the extreme scenario of a new species caused by changes on a human being's genome would *not* necessarily introduce a non-human being: although it is debatable whether genetic interventions could produce another species, the evolutionary view of species membership that DeGrazia is arguing for includes the descendants of a given species within the species' boundary.[79]

How biotechnological enhancement provides real benefits for its users has been a major topic for writers intellectually or institutionally close to Bostrom for at least a decade. Sandberg, for example, has provided a detailed analysis of the means and ends of cognitive enhancement.[80] Particular benefits expected from biotechnological enhancement are the improvement of attention, reduction of tiredness, improvement of memory and memory retention, better performance in spatial planning, reduction of reaction time, improved learning, improved creativity etc.

---

[75] DeGrazia 2005: 275.
[76] Ibid.: 275.
[77] Ibid.: 276.
[78] Ibid.: 277.
[79] Cf. ibid.: 278.
[80] Cf. Sandberg 2011.

Sandberg, Julian Savulescu and others explored the use of biotechnological enhancement for the promotion[81] and inhibition[82] of love. They suggest that biotechnological interventions can be used to facilitate fidelity, to improve pair bonding where desired or to reduce such bonding in toxic relationships.

Some of these authors have turned the individual benefit into a definiens of human enhancement by providing the above-mentioned welfarist definition of enhancement.[83] According to this definition, an increase in the chances of leading a good life turns a biotechnological intervention into an enhancement. A good life is the classical goal pursued for its own sake.

5.1.1.2 Means of leading an authentic life

Authenticity denotes states in which the original convictions and wishes of people are expressed in their thoughts and actions. In contrast, lack of authenticity is understood as a distortion of this original self-expression and as alienation from one's own goals. As a moral ideal, authenticity demands that each person finds and implements his or her own original form of expression and way of life.

Biotechnological enhancements have been identified as possible means of overcoming sources of inauthenticity in an individual life. Such a potential has especially been claimed for antidepressants, as vividly demonstrated by Peter Kramer who presents the case of his patient Tess. Tess is given Prozac after an older antidepressant had already lifted her beyond the standard criteria of depression but at the cost of serious side-effects. Kramer describes the change brought about by Prozac as follows:

»I have never seen a person's social life reshaped so rapidly and dramatically. Low self-worth, competitiveness, jealousy, poor interpersonal skills, shyness, fear of intimacy—the usual causes of social awkwardness—are so deeply ingrained and so difficult to influence that ordinarily change comes gradually if at all. But Tess blossomed all at once.«[84]

In her own perception, Tess is enabled to be who she really is and to live an authentic life by the means of Prozac. Provided inauthenticity is a kind of harm and authenticity a kind of good, this is another source for positive consequentialist evaluation of biotechnological enhancement.[85]

---

[81] Cf. Savulescu / Sandberg 2008.
[82] Cf. Earp et al. 2013.
[83] Cf. Savulescu / Sandberg / Kahane 2011.
[84] Kramer 1994: 8.
[85] Cf. ibid.; DeGrazia 2000; id. 2005.

Initially, arguments from authenticity have been employed *against enhancement,* supporting the claim that enhancement undermines authenticity.[86] This has been the original worry uttered by Carl Elliott in his thought-provoking *The tyranny of happiness* (1998). He exposes a complex dialectic of enhancement as a tool in the pursuit of happiness, a cultural norm of pursuing one's happiness which has assumed obligatory character, and the risk of glossing over weighty reasons for being unhappy by biotechnological means.

This enhancement-critical challenge has been answered by DeGrazia[87], who explored whether there are principled reasons making it impossible to use biotechnological interventions for the pursuit of an authentic life. DeGrazia's main claim is a negative one, namely that there are no such principled reasons against biotechnological enhancements. The positive support for his claim that enhancement can be a tool for an authentic life is predominantly found in his examples. His main example introduces a person who has a non-pathological degree of compulsiveness and feels like she is therefore not able to pursue the way of life she would otherwise prefer. If she judges a way of life that has previous to her taking Prozac been unavailable to her as what would most authentically be hers, and given further that biotechnological methods can be an authentic way to pursue this way of life, there seems to be no possible instance which could correct her judgement. A philosopher who claims that it is inauthentic for this particular person to pursue a way of life by biotechnological means assumes for herself or himself to be a better judge of another person's life. This would be a form of strong paternalism, which finds few serious adherents in contemporary ethics. Thus, if no principled reasons can be found against biomedical enhancement as a tool for authenticity and one wants to shun away from strong paternalism, the potential for critique to pursuing a chosen way of life with the help of technological enhancement seems to be exhausted.

Parens has revived a traditional core distinction in conceptions of authenticity, one referring to self-determined choice of options, the other to an unfolding of a person's original characteristics. These two understandings of the term make for two different frameworks for thought about one's own good life, creativity, and gratefulness. Biotechnological enhancement has, previous to Parens' analysis, typically been associated with what he came to call the *framework of creativity*[88], i. e. a frame of mind

---

[86] Cf. Chatterjee 2004; Elliott 1998.
[87] DeGrazia 2000: 35. Cf. also Bublitz / Merkel 2009: 372.
[88] Cf. Parens 2005.

oriented towards self-modification and self-perfection. But as Neil Levy has pointed out, neuroenhancement of mood and cognition can be regarded as supportive of a person's authenticity regardless of the respective concept of authenticity used.[89] On the self-creation view of authenticity, the use of biotechnological enhancement is a tool for personal ›reinvention‹. On the self-discovery view the same interventions can be interpreted as a process in which the individual's outer expression is brought into agreement with »who we most deeply are«.[90] Neuroenhancement procedures would thus merely be a means of expressing an existing personality core.[91] In summary, there seems to be a strong case for considering biotechnological enhancement as a possible means for an authentic life.

5.1.1.3 _Support of character and virtue development_
In response to the debate about authenticity, authors with a background in virtue ethics discussed by which means persons should develop their character or virtues in order to live a good life. Amongst these authors, those who took a liberal view often argued ex negativo, i.e. refuted the contributions critical of enhancement by restrictive authors. On the one hand, restrictive approaches like those of Elliott or Michael Sandel typically argue for an alteration of a person's given natural gifts by practice and learning of virtues within social practices alone—and therefore criticize what they consider unnatural enhancement-shortcuts in any self-creation project.[92] Proponents of enhancement, on the other hand, criticize the lack of clarity, precision, and adequacy of the notions ›true self‹ and ›authenticity‹ as well as the restrictive concepts of virtue and a good human life. Felicitas Kraemer diagnosed that »there is a widely held intuition that an artificial means will always lead to an inauthentic result.«[93] This is perhaps why, for the most part, virtue ethical contributions have been criticizing enhancement, especially neuroenhancement.[94] The few virtue ethical arguments in favour of enhancement mainly consist of criticisms on strong opponent versions stressing their problematic and demanding presuppositions[95], or in analyzing the concept of virtues.[96] They do not

---

[89] Cf. Levy 2011: 312.
[90] Ibid.: 317.
[91] For a reply cf. Erler 2012. For an overview cf. id. 2014.
[92] For a critical analysis of Sandel's _The case against perfection_ (2007), cf. ter Meulen 2019.
[93] Kraemer 2011: 51.
[94] Cf. also section 5.1.2.6 (»Limits to the development of character and virtues«).
[95] Cf. e.g. DeGrazia 2000: 35f.
[96] Cf. e.g. Schermer 2008: 363.

merely show that enhancement methods can be compatible with virtue ethical accounts of authenticity and a good human life. Beyond that, they try to establish that either there is nothing like an essential human nature and identity, or that at least the latter are not at risk. Interestingly enough, none of the proponents deny the importance of safety and thoughtfulness considering the usage of an optional use of neuroenhancers in non-medical contexts. However, they suggest that neuroenhancement must not be seen as necessarily detrimental to character, practice of virtue, or the human life form as it might actually simplify the access to or implementation of a better and more virtuous life.

The class of virtue ethical arguments is often unjustifiably omitted in the general neuroenhancement debate. In addition, the influence of virtue ethical thought seems to be growing in recent years. This is why we summarize the supporting arguments as well as the counterarguments from a virtue ethical point of view more comprehensively for the first time.

The virtue of self-creation
It was DeGrazia who first argued that the pessimism of restrictive views is exaggerated when they expect that the use of biotechnological enhancement will result in a decay of character and thus a person's life. He even seems to argue for the opposite claim, namely that biotechnological enhancement can positively shape a person's ability for self-creation. According to him, self-creation is considered to be an ability which can be developed. To support this claim, he argues that self-creation cannot be seen as entirely independent of our agency, but must rather be understood as a process of conscious and deliberate shaping of personality, character, or life direction which depends on the self-conception or self-narration a person considers to be most important: »who we are has everything to do with what we value.«[97]

In light of this, he states that enhancement methods can indeed provide shortcuts to reaching certain goals and facilitate the process of self-creation. They constitute one means (among others) of authentic self-creation because »values and self-conception are the basis for the chosen means.«[98] Thus, the process of self-creation and overcoming certain emotional or personal struggles that hinder this process are to be seen as powerful expressions of agency.[99] These processes can be facilitated by neuroenhancement.

---

[97] DeGrazia 2000: 37.
[98] Ibid.: 38.
[99] Cf. ibid.: 39.

In a more recent contribution, DeGrazia explicitly shows that moral bioenhancement does not pose a »significant across-the-board thread to freedom«[100] since being a subject of moral bioenhancement is itself an individual's choice and therefore an expression of agency.

The virtue of self-discipline

Maartje Schermer provides another argument exposing the shortcut-argument given by restrictive views according to which the development of character and virtues can only be achieved by effort, struggle, pain, patience, and practice over a longer period of time and that thus enhancement is detrimental to that process: the fact that suffering *sometimes* enables learning and wisdom does not imply that it is *necessarily* so, since »not all suffering involves learning or promotes wisdom. Suffering can make people rather nasty and unpleasant—it is not always ›purifying‹ or ›enriching‹.«[101]

Even if it would be the case that certain enhancement technologies have detrimental effects on an individual's character, it would probably only affect certain aspects of character since virtues like »justice, wisdom, humanity or transcendence appear to be less vulnerable to the use of enhancers.«[102] Moreover, Schermer highlights that there are some basic virtues with context-sensitive expression and interpretation which can change with time and culture and can be practiced in various different ways through different activities. This would not only imply that there is »plenty of opportunity to practise [sic!] and cultivate the main virtues«[103], but it is also another argument showing that the restrictive position's worry about the corrosion of character seem to be exaggerated.

In her positive argument, Schermer employs a concept of self-discipline which is much closer to a skill-model of this virtue. This contrasts starkly to the strength- or endurance-model of self-discipline employed by several of the more restrictive authors such as Leon Kass and the President's Council. She stresses that »[i]t is better to put one's energy and virtues into activities that deserve it, rather than into activities whose goals can be reached in easier ways«[104] for it would be easily disregarded that »while technologies can indeed inhibit certain behaviour, they also invite others« with their »enabling, amplifying, or innovative effects.«[105]

---

[100] DeGrazia 2013: 6.
[101] Schermer 2008: 359.
[102] Ibid.: 357.
[103] Ibid.: 358.
[104] Ibid.
[105] Ibid.: 362.

Schermer argues that enhancement technologies cannot merely be evaluated according to their effect on focal practice—i. e. dynamic forms of engagement with the world that sponsor discipline, skill, and are exercised in a unity of achievement and enjoyment having some tradition, structure, and rhythm. In addition, it must be taken into account whether they reduce or disrupt the obtainment of goods and forms of excellence.[106]

Facilitating the acquisition of virtue & overcoming biology

A similar approach like those of DeGrazia and Schermer, showing that enhancement can facilitate the acquisition of virtue, is given by Barbro Fröding: »[s]ome cognitive enhancements might not only be seen as neutral from a virtue perspective but indeed as facilitating, for example, the habituation process.«[107] She states that neuroenhancement could enable people to »become more virtuous« by overcoming their »biological makeup« which is taken to be the »worst enemy in the quest for the good life.«[108] Fröding explains more specifically *why* and *how* enhancement could facilitate the development of moral and epistemic virtues: our biological nature gives us natural constraints that fail to develop moral and epistemic virtues, which can only be overcome through medical or technical enhancement methods and by internalizing virtues more successfully.[109] Since cognitive enhancements are »unlikely to mimic all the worthwhile aspects of the virtuous life«[110], we also need the experience of exercising them for »actual process [that] is valuable by itself.«[111] Taking practice as a serious part in the achievement of virtues is clearly in line with the standard version of virtue ethics.[112] Fröding also mentions that we could neither fully develop virtues on our own, nor only through enhancement. In the former case, we would be hindered by natural constraints; in the latter case, we would not have the practice and wisdom which are also necessary to develop virtues. Only both forms of achievement taken together could lead us to a good life. In order to evaluate

---

[106] Cf. Schermer 2008: 361 ff.

[107] Fröding 2011: 231.

[108] Ibid.

[109] Cf. ibid.: 224.

[110] Ibid.: 229.

[111] Ibid.: 230.

[112] For a more in-depth discussion of the requirements and some historical remarks of virtue ethical arguments especially linked to the enhancement debate cf. Heinrichs / Stake 2019. For an overall introduction to virtue ethics cf. e. g. Hursthouse / Pettigrove 2016.

which enhancement methods could be good or bad, Fröding suggests an evaluation on the basis of how well they contribute to a good life, especially considering the key aspects of »safety, voluntariness, autonomy and informed consent, fairness and transparency«.[113]

A similar thought can be found in Kraemer (2011) who argues that emotional authenticity is to be regarded as a phenomenal quality based on which it is possible to recognize and identify feelings according to three standards of emotion: the authenticity standard, the rationality standard, and the coherence standard. She concludes that although some neuroenhancers do not always meet all the standards, e.g. Prozac, »[t]here are *artificially* induced *authentic* emotional states. And vice versa, there are *naturally* engendered emotions that turn out to be *inauthentic*.«[114]

Necessary for constitution of cognitive virtues (e. g. autonomy)

Last but not least, the recent approach of J. Adam Carter defends that »even some extreme kinds of cognitive enhancement might be not merely compatible with, but constitutive of, virtuous intellectual autonomy.«[115] Carter emphasizes that the virtuous autonomous agent must already rely on others and therefore »outsource cognitive tasks as a means to gaining knowledge and other epistemic goods, *up until the point that doing so would be at the expense of her own capacity for self-direction.*«[116] Moreover, he is inspired by the »parity principle«, firstly introduced by Andy Clark and David Chalmers[117] and accepts that something should count as a part of cognitive processes if it has the same functional role, the same accessibility as a person's biological brain. As such it is part of the person's character, falls under the ownership conditions and can play a role in belief formation, i.e. can be appreciated as reliable.[118] Following this train of thought, the question whether new enhancement technologies are to be integrated would not be a matter of what we are relying on or why we are depending on it, but it rather would matter *how* we are depending on it, which »remains largely in our own hands.«[119] This means that the threat of an undermined intellectual autonomy would not be given because of the use or application of enhancements but rather because of the lack of

---

[113] Fröding 2011: 232.
[114] Kraemer 2011: 63.
[115] Carter 2017: 2.
[116] Ibid.: 4.
[117] Cf. Clark / Chalmers 1998.
[118] Carter 2017: 14.
[119] Ibid.: 22.

their suitable cognitive integration, which is firstly a case of awareness and secondly a case of learning.[120]

5.1.2 Counterarguments

5.1.2.1 *Adverse (and long-term) effects*

The most straightforward consequentialist argument against enhancement lists the harms of biotechnological interventions. Should they outweigh the benefits, as several authors suggest, this would be a conclusive reason against their use. The mere fact that there are such harms, however, is not conclusive, although otherwise suggested by some authors.[121] The evaluation of biotechnological enhancements gets more complicated if they are just one among several possible means towards a specific end. If there are multiple means, the analysis of adverse effects will have to be a comparative one. If, for example, rigorous physical training and anabolic steroids could produce the same effect, the effort and side effects (adverse and positive) of both methods must be compared. Non-biotechnological means exist for several enhancement projects, including projects typically pursued with neuro-active biotechnologies. And while the side-effects of biotechnological enhancements have meanwhile been investigated in some detail[122], those of non-technological means typically are not mentioned in the literature. One exception can be found in Levy's comparison of the use of Ritalin and the reduction of class sizes in order to promote educational success.[123]

One of the more widely discussed forms of adverse effects especially of neuropharmacological enhancements is the risk of addiction. There have been two ongoing strands in the debate, one from a clinically dominated perspective raising awareness for this specific risk[124], the other from a more theoretical perspective engaging with the concept ›addiction‹ and its validity as a nosological entity or construct.[125] The latter strand of the debate revolves around the etiology of addictive phenomena and whether they are to be considered a dysfunctional learning process or a disease.

---

[120] Cf. Carter 2017: 19.
[121] Cf. Douglas 2015.
[122] Cf. Repantis et al. 2009; Repantis / Laisney / Heuser 2010; Repantis et al. 2010; Smith / Farah 2011; Ilieva / Boland / Farah 2013.
[123] Cf. Levy 2007. Another direct comparison like the development of honours programmes to other forms of enhancement can be found in Olthof et al. 2013.
[124] Cf. Lieb 2010.
[125] Cf. Carter et al. 2011. Cf. also the Special Issue »Addiction Neuroscience« of *Neuroethics*.

A non-pathological but still devastating form of dependence can be generated via overreliance on biotechnological means. Persons relying on such means can come to doubt their unsupported capacity for dealing with life's obstacles, and thereby in fact lose a part of this capacity.[126]

It has repeatedly been claimed that the risk-benefit analysis for therapeutic intervention and for enhancing intervention will produce different results in most of the cases. Therapeutic value is thought to outweigh adverse effects in more cases than enhancement effects. While there is little rationale to value welfare gained by therapeutic measures higher than that gained by biotechnological enhancement, there seems to be a good reasons why therapeutic interventions often have a better risk-benefit ratio. In the case of therapeutic decisions there typically is a higher cost of omission. The cost of inaction in therapeutic contexts often, if not always, is a further deterioration of health, while there is normally no comparable cost in decisions for or against biotechnological enhancement.

5.1.2.2 _Fraudulent happiness_

The positive consequentialist argument for biotechnological enhancement as described above claims that there are individual benefits to be gained. Enhancements carry promises of individual welfare gains. There are two common counters to this argument starting from the concept of fraudulent happiness.

The first counter insists that the positive argument itself does not even get off the ground because the welfare gains in question are only pretence. The second counter accepts that there are welfare gains from biotechnological enhancement but suggests that these are inferior to welfare from other sources and thus carry the risk of replacing superior by inferior sources of welfare. These arguments have come to be known under the title of ›fraudulent happiness arguments‹. The term has been taken up from the President's Council on Bioethics Report, which claims:

»Yet a fraudulent happiness is just what the pharmacological management of our mental lives threatens to confer upon us.«[127]

The two issues associated with fraudulent happiness in the President's Council Report are 1) that »an unchecked power to [...] brighten moods, and alter our emotional dispositions could imperil our capacity to form a strong and coherent personal identity«[128], and second that »by discon-

---

[126] Cf. Moesgen / Klein 2015: 69.
[127] President's Council of Bioethics (U.S.) 2003: 210.
[128] Ibid.: 212. This challenge has been addressed in Krämer 2011.

necting our mood [...] from what we do and experience, the new drugs could jeopardize the fitness and truthfulness of how we live and what we feel«.[129] The first of these two issues is related to questions of authentic personality and will thus be discussed in the section below. The second one relates to what has been called a ›reality constraint‹. Happiness is, according to this thought, valuable only if it derives from a person's activities.[130] Happiness caused by other means or by an activity in combination with other means such as biotechnological intervention is, in contrast, to be considered fraudulent. As Birgit Beck and Barbara Stroop argue, this criticism of biotechnological enhancement as producing only fraudulent happiness requires a strong objective theory of happiness.[131] Even then it is not clear whether all uses of biotechnological mood enhancers fall prey to a criticism based on the objective activity-based conception of happiness. As some of the examples most often used in the literature show, biotechnological enhancement can be used in order to be able to participate in certain activities in the appropriate mood. Happiness is taken to be the result of these activities and not the outcome of the use of biotechnological enhancement directly. One such standard example used for instance by David Wasserman and S. Matthew Liao[132] as well as Liao and Rebecca Roache[133] is that of a person who wants to use a psychoactive substance in order to be able to cheerfully participate in a celebration. If the analysis provided by the authors is correct, the fraudulent happiness argument can successfully target the pursuit of elevated or ecstatic mood by means of psychoactives, i. e. a passive drug high, but only few others forms of biotechnological enhancement.

5.1.2.3 *Negative impact of enhanced traits*

Some authors have claimed that not merely the welfare promises, but also the promises of improved capacities are ridden with difficulties. This claim also comes in two variants: the first denies that biotechnological enhancement will result in improved capacities, the second one points out that improvements via biotechnological means either carry unwanted side effects or are otherwise inferior to other possible improvements or even to the status quo. The claim that biotechnological enhancement does not result in improved capacities and that the side-effects are predomi-

---

[129] President's Council of Bioethics (U.S.) 2003: 213. For a detailed discussion about this issue cf. Kahane 2011.
[130] Cf. ibid.: 265.
[131] Cf. Beck / Stroop 2015.
[132] Cf. Wasserman / Liao 2008.
[133] Cf. Liao / Roache 2011.

nant has already been covered in the above discussion. However, it is equally claimed that possible improvements will not live up to their promise for some other reason. One of the more vivid examples has been brought into the debate by Liao and Sandberg. They refer to the case of Alexander Luria, who had extreme memory recall abilities. However, he often was unable to use these abilities for action guidance. Liao and Sandberg point out that an improvement of memory can be detrimental to daily life at the same time.[134] A similar effect has already been pointed out for the case of enhancement via memory modulation, which might seriously and maybe adversely affect the development of a person's character traits.[135]

5.1.2.4   *Loss of authenticity*

As mentioned above, the idea that biotechnological enhancement might be detrimental to authenticity has preceded the suggestion that it could be a tool in the pursuit of an authentic life.[136] Although this idea has found a plethora of replies, it has been suggested by fewer authors than one would expect. In the President's Council's Report it is suspected that any biotechnological enhancement can endanger the development of a person's character traits by loosening the link between that person's biological structure, her social upbringing, her experiences, and her emotional and cognitive reactions to the former. The core idea seems to be that persons best develop their character by engaging with their surroundings without any recourse to biotechnological or other artificial means beyond therapy.[137] The Council's suggestion has—amongst others—been criticised for its identification of artificiality and inauthenticity[138], its essentialism[139], and its static conception of character.[140] The more complex argument presented by Elliot suggests that the pursuit of happiness via biotechnological interventions can be experienced as a strong cultural imperative, and following this imperative can result in a loss of authenticity.[141] Later contributions highlight the effect of biotechnological interventions on a person's qualitative personality as conceptualised by a narrative theory of personal identity. As mentioned above, Lavazza

---

[134] Cf. Liao / Sandberg 2008: 89.
[135] Cf. President's Council of Bioethics (U.S.) 2003; Lavazza 2018a.
[136] Cf. section 5.1.1.2 (»Means of leading an authentic life«).
[137] Cf. President's Council of Bioethics (U.S.) 2003: 280 ff.
[138] Cf. Kraemer 2011.
[139] Cf. Levy 2011.
[140] Cf. Bublitz / Merkel 2009.
[141] Cf. Elliott 1998.

describes the potential of memory modification to affect a person's narrative identity.[142]

There is a surprising number of contributions which discuss the effect of Deep Brain Stimulation (DBS) on the patient's authenticity as a reason against the use of DBS for enhancement.[143] Pugh and colleagues for example explicitly connect their account of DBS effects on authenticity to the enhancement debate[144]. Most authors in the debate, however, accept that procedures as invasive as DBS will become candidates for enhancement use only in a rather remote future. As a consequence, arguments concerning the effect of DBS on authenticity are mostly transferred to other, more proximal biotechnological enhancements by analogy.

5.1.2.5 *Human Nature and its components*

Amongst the most intensively debated arguments concerning enhancement are those building on the concept of human nature.[145] One of the key starting points in this regard is the repeatedly mentioned President's Council on Bioethics. According to the Council, »the human body and mind, highly complex and delicately balanced, as the result of eons of gradual and exacting evolution, are almost certainly at risk from any ill-considered attempt at improvement.«[146] In this passage, the Council can be read as claiming that human nature is already in an optimal condition and is, therefore, not in need of any cognitive or other forms of enhancement.

Advocates of permissive positions have given various responses to this ›optimal nature‹-argument. To begin with, the Council was accused of committing all kinds of logical mistakes, first and foremost, the famous Is-ought-fallacy[147] because their argument draws normative conclusions, namely that the natural status quo is the human optimum and should not be modified, from a descriptive interpretation of human nature as shaped by evolutionary processes. A further critique tackles the Council's understanding of evolution. According to Buchanan, the Council supposes that

---

[142] That enhancement might risk authenticity has also been suggested by Bolt 2007 and Berghmans et al. 2011.
[143] Empirical evidence for such an effect is presented in De Haan et al. 2017.
[144] Cf. Pugh / Maslen / Savulescu 2017. This article makes use of a diachronic account of authenticity, which contrasts with a synchronic understanding of authenticity is developed by Sven Nyholm and Elizabeth O'Neill. Cf. Nyholm / O'Neill 2016; id. 2017.
[145] For an insightful analysis of the function of the concept in the debate cf. Buchanan 2009b.
[146] President's Council of Bioethics (U.S.) 2003: 287.
[147] For an overview of the discussion cf. Cerullo 2009; Green 2010.

evolution is a master engineer who makes her creation a »stable, completed masterpiece that can only be ruined by any human attempt to improve it.«[148] For Buchanan, this sounds like an unsatisfactory re-enchantment of nature that brings ancient natural teleology back into today's philosophical business.

Setting aside these scientific and metaphysical issues, there is also a lingering normative challenge to the ›optimal-nature‹-argument. Why should we see our human nature—as the Council does—as »delicately balanced« in the first place? Some permissive positions point to the fact that our natural set-up as seems to be at least locally defective and intuitively more credible form the perspective of our everyday life practice.[149] For some the situation looks even worse as they think of our human nature as not only locally, but generally flawed. For instance, some have argued—in a Kantian spirit—that human nature is morally fragile and tends to corruption so that enhancement is an indirect duty to oneself.[150] From these perspectives, claiming that human nature is already optimal is at best an unjustified bias towards the status quo which disregards the problems that human nature produces for itself and the environment.[151] So why still stick to the claim that human nature should be preserved? At this dialectical point, the advocate of the restrictive position is forced to propose an argument that does not solely assume the intuitive preferability of the current state of human nature. He must come up with an idea *which* concrete aspects of human nature are in danger and *why* that threat justifies a ban of enhancement. Some of the options explored in the literature will be discussed in the following.

Autonomy as a precondition of the moral community

A widely discussed suggestion was brought forward by Juergen Habermas.[152] He claims that an essential part of human nature consists in having a self-image as equally free, self-legislating beings. For Habermas, this is not only an important fact about the *conditio humana*, but also constitutes a conceptual precondition for humans to participate in a moral community, even more so one ruled by equality and human rights. Thus, if

---

[148] Buchanan 2011: 156.

[149] The locus classicus for this point is John Stuart Mill in his famous description of nature: »This brief survey is amply sufficient to prove that the duty of man is the same in respect to his own nature as in respect to the nature of all other things, namely not to follow but to amend it« (Mill 1969: 397).

[150] Cf. Bauer 2018.

[151] Cf. Bostrom / Ord 2006.

[152] For the core formulation of the argument cf. Habermas 2003.

something threatens our understanding as equal, autonomous persons, it also threatens the basis of the moral community and of democratic society as a whole. According to Habermas, the liberal eugenics of human enhancement does exactly this. He provides several reasons for his claim, most of which are empirical and support a consequentialist case against liberal eugenics.[153] However, there is also at least one deontological reason which can be called the *argument from prenatality*.[154] The argument rests on the idea that in order to be an autonomous person, a point of reference is required »which goes back beyond the lines of tradition and the contexts of interaction«[155], namely a socially unaffected prenatal point. Only if some remote beginning of her natural endowment is unaffected by social forces, a person can understand herself as the source and author of actions. Accordingly, if a child's prenatal abilities or traits are changed by enhancement, then that child will not be able to conceive of himself as having an identity beyond that which is determined by his socialization. But this also implies that the autonomous self-image of the individual who is prenatally enhanced would »slip away«, as Habermas claims.[156] The individual could not understand him- or herself as an autonomous agent, which not only results in a mistreatment of his or her own nature, but also undermines the enhanced individual's ability to regard him- or herself as member of a moral community of equals. As this moral affiliation is the core of human morality according to Habermas' own theory of ethics, liberal eugenics endangers the very ethics of the species.

Dignity and self-worth
A further aspect of human nature that has been discussed in the enhancement debate is the moral worth or dignity of the enhanced agent. The underlying worry can be summarized in the following way: The use of enhancement techniques affects key features of human nature that are responsible for generating moral worth and dignity so that the enhanced individual either fails to have dignity or has less dignity than unenhanced individuals. There are different views of what exactly constitutes dignity or moral worth. Thus, Francis Fukuyama states that it is a ›factor x‹ which is not in need of further analysis.[157] For others, the constitutive

---

[153] For a careful consideration cf. Pugh 2015.
[154] Habermas explicitly refers to Hannah Arendt's idea of natality in this context.
[155] Habermas 2003: 59.
[156] Ibid.: 60.
[157] Cf. Fukuyama 2002: 149 ff.

factor is rationality[158], a special sort of »naturalness«[159], or even some divine property conferred by a creator.[160]

Character and virtue

A further component of human nature that some find worth exploring are specific attitudes or character traits. Sandel advances an argument that can be seen as a version of this line of reasoning by focusing on the virtue of humility.[161] Linking back to his criticism of liberalism in political philosophy, Sandel interprets human societies as having a drive to master and control nature, which is taken to the extreme in human enhancement. For Sandel, this drive threatens to result in a hyperagency that loses the appreciation for natural features to be cherished as they are. What he advocates is an attitude of humility which includes an »openness to the unbidden«.[162] For Sandel, this does not necessarily include the theistic belief in the goodness and preservation of God's creation. Rather, he thinks that the value of giftedness can be understood in secular terms, namely as an act of humility (humbly accepting the cards one has been dealt) that is an essential feature of human nature.[163]

Way of being

Another facet of human nature that has been discussed in the literature is the special relation the species has to its environment or even the whole of the universe. A version of this idea is developed by Michael Hauskeller who builds on the concept of humility introduced by Sandel.[164] Hauskeller carefully unpacks the notion of humility and observes that the crucial aspect of human nature is not a character trait but a »way of being«[165] that normatively grounds it. He argues that by humbly appreciating the giftedness of our natural abilities we create a bond between us and the rest of the world. We generate a feeling of »being at home in the world«[166] because we recognize ourselves as part of a comprehensive whole. For Hauskeller, this mode of being is threatened by enhancement since its

---

[158] Cf. Lee / George 2008.

[159] Cf. Siep 2004; Sturma 2019.

[160] Cf. Meilaender 2008: 264.

[161] Cf. Sandel 2007: chapter 5.

[162] Sandel 2007: 45.

[163] For virtue ethical arguments cf. also section 5.1.2.6 (»Limits to the development of character and virtues«).

[164] Cf. Hauskeller 2011.

[165] Ibid.: 76.

[166] Ibid.: 74.

underlying drive to mastery takes our nature as something that has to be improved and thus leads to a mode of being which can be best described as personal alienation and cosmic homelessness.

The human nature argument and its critics

There are several critical replies that have been submitted against each of these suggestions. However, a locus classicus in the debate are the considerations of Buchanan which are spread and developed across his writings.[167] In its most basic version, Buchanan seems to formulate a dilemma for all advocates of the ›human nature‹-argument: either the term »human nature« is used as a mere placeholder and can be dropped for a more precise terminology or else it leads to what Buchanan calls »normative essentialism«, a position which claims that a fixed feature (or set of features) of human nature is suited to derive moral norms from.[168] Either way, according to Buchanan this puts the advocate of the ›human nature‹-argument in a very unsettling situation. However, there have been various rejoinders, followed by re-rejoinders and re-re-rejoinders.[169] The debate literally fills bookstores, ranging from methodological issues to epistemological or metaphysical challenges, and is still not settled.[170]

5.1.2.6 *Limits to the development of character and virtues*

Traditionally, arguments that rely heavily on character and virtues and its development are considered in the context of virtue ethics. As all classical concepts of virtue ethics aim to be holistic concepts for the good human life—most of all by the implementation and praxis of virtues (among other important preconditions)—, they are linked to concepts of an ideal human life and its natural talents and characteristics that were briefly introduced in the previous section.[171] In the human strife for excellent behaviour, it is important to understand that from a virtue ethical point of view, human beings learn to be virtuous through both practice of the virtues and the intellectual understanding of what is valuable. The refer-

---

[167] For this argument cf. Buchanan 2009b.

[168] Cf. ibid. This is a very general argument against all versions of the human nature argument. It is noteworthy though, that Buchanan unpacks almost all of the arguments mentioned above and carefully examines their plausibility case by case. As an example, cf. his exploration of the autonomy argument by Habermas which seems not been backed up by »sound reasoning«. Cf. Buchanan 2011: 6.

[169] For an overview cf. Lewens 2012; Groll / Lott 2015; Pugh / Kahane / Savulescu 2016.

[170] For a more detailed analysis of the discussion cf. Rüther / Heinrichs 2019.

[171] Whether a concept of a natural self or natural characteristics is necessary for a virtue ethical concept is an open question since it depends on the notion of human nature. Cf. also section 5.1.2.5 (»Human nature and its components«).

ence to character forms an essential part of virtue ethics in any attempt to justify right actions.[172] But what could be wrong with neuroenhancement according to a virtue ethical framework?

Inauthenticity, lack of ownership and unnatural development of character
One of the classic counterarguments in the debate is provided by Kass who claims that human beings could not »really own the transformations nor experience them as genuinely«[173] when they rely on enhancement technologies. Consequently, the use of such technologies leads to a form of inauthenticity. Therefore, Kass considers enhancement as an ethically dubious or unacceptable means to overcome natural limitations of human beings who »master, control, and even transform one's own given nature«.[174] So-called *improvements* by enhancement methods could produce changes in the very core of humanness, »disrupting the normal character, [...] skip[ping] the realm of intelligible meaning« so that »we cannot really own the transformations nor experience them as genuinely ours.«[175] Kass has an Aristotelian understanding of the good and flourishing human life as one where »the engaged and energetic being-at-work of what nature uniquely gave to us is what we need to treasure and defend. All other perfection is at best a passing illusion, at worst a Faustian bargain that will cost us our full and flourishing humanity.«[176] This specific understanding of ›flourishing‹ presupposes that a good human life has to be naturally given, i. e. born and developed without artificial means, whatever they are. Accordingly, any enhancement method that alters what is naturally given would have to be understood as an inauthentic means. This ›argument of inauthenticity‹ has been reiterated in different versions by other opponents of neuroenhancement.[177] They all share the view that any kind of enhancement technology is prima facie confronted with the accusation to be an unnatural means that can only lead to inauthentic results, which are therefore not compatible with the original pursuit. In this context, authors often make use of an intuitive, if highly contested,

---

[172] Considering the criterion of rightness explained by Rosalind Hursthouse, an action is right if and only if it is what an agent with a virtuous character would do in the same circumstances not solely oriented on outcomes or social rules. This is a typical standpoint of the *generalists*. In contrast, the *particularists* do not consider a perfect ideal, but rather emphasize the human ability to recognize what is morally good by trained perception. Cf. Hursthouse 1996: 22.

[173] Kass 2003: 24. Cf. for a similar line of reasoning Sturma 2019: 146.

[174] Kass 2003: 17.

[175] Ibid.: 24.

[176] Ibid.: 28.

[177] For more examples cf. section 5.1.2.4 (»Loss of authenticity«).

differentiation between ›natural‹ and ›artificial‹/›unnatural‹ as well as the presupposition that natural means are generally better than unnatural ones. This suggests that we are able to recognize and know the meaning of ›the real nature‹ or ›essential nature‹ of a situation, thing, or individual. Strong versions of this type of argument for restrictive approaches are also endorsed by Charles Taylor[178], Alasdair MacIntyre[179], or Sandel[180]. They are linked to a notion of a true individual self.[181]

The burden of responsibility

Another important argument against enhancement technologies that has also been presented by Sandel builds on the fear of altering the agent's autonomy. According to Sandel, autonomy matures by appropriate praxis within a social community.[182] His main argument targets social solidarity that could only be fostered if the individual's natural talents are seen as a matter of good fortune. Once individuals start to alter themselves by technological means, social solidarity would be undermined to the effect that the natural talents of those individuals will no longer be the primary source of their own successes in life, but will rather depend on their undertaking technological enhancements. This would affect, if not diminish, the individual sense of responsibility as well as a broad consensus on justice.

»If bioengineering made the myth of the ›self-made man‹ come true, it would be difficult to view our talents as gifts for which we are indebted, rather than as achievements for which we are responsible. This would transform three key features of our moral landscape: humility, responsibility, and solidarity.«[183]

Interestingly enough and contrary to the common claim that enhancement would lead to *less* responsibility, Sandel worries that responsibility could expand to »daunting proportions« since we would »attribute less to chance and more to choice.«[184] According to Sandel, »one of the blessings of seeing ourselves as creatures of nature, God, or fortune is that we are not wholly responsible for the way we are. The more we become masters

---

[178] Cf. Taylor 1991.
[179] Cf. MacIntyre 2007.
[180] Cf. Sandel 2012.
[181] Cf. also the arguments relying on the concept of human nature in section 5.1.2.5 (»Human nature and its components«).
[182] Cf. Sandel 2012. Cf. also the character and virtue argument by Sandel in section 5.1.2.5 (»Human nature and its components«).
[183] Sandel 2012: 102. Cf. also Orlebeke Caldera 2008.
[184] Sandel 2012: 102.

of our genetic endowments, the greater the burden we bear for the talents we have and the way we perform.«[185]

Sandel continues to argue that participation in social practices requires specific and general virtues.[186] The core general virtue in this regard is the capacity for judgement. This capacity of judgement (*phronēsis*) is a necessary precondition for exercising any other character virtue.[187] Implementing enhancement methods would not only threaten an important form of socially embedded practice, but also undermine the capacity of judgment. This last argument can already be found in Elliott[188] and later in Andreas Vieth who specifically argues that every enhancing manipulation of the self transforms natural human individuals into cyborgs. Vieth considers this transformation to be morally problematic since it is not a »natural change« and at odds with the concept of justice which is deeply embedded in common human practice of »normal social discourse«.[189] Since enhancement could lead to a lack of practice and thus to a lack of character virtues, a loss of authenticity, and lack of autonomy, it might not only alter the individual, but also threaten society as a whole.

Creating epistemic harm

Regarding intellectual virtues and responsibility, Lubomira Radoilska argues that even if the outcomes of an epistemic action, i. e. an action used to change the world in order to gain information or simplify a problem-solving task[190], with or without enhancement are nearly identical, any form of enhancement, especially neuroenhancement, leads to some extent to epistemic harm, such as second-hand knowledge and self-deception. This is due to the fact that epistemic outcomes would not be fully creditable to the agent »and in this sense do not constitute an unambiguous epistemic achievement« for which the agent could consequently not be held fully responsible.[191] This »epistemic harm« or »partial loss of epistemic credit« would already be »instigated by the failure to appreciate intel-

---

[185] Sandel 2012: 103.
[186] In this vain he follows MacIntyre 2007: 150.
[187] Whereas intellectual virtues can be acquired by teaching, the virtues of character can only be acquired through habitual practice. Nevertheless, both sorts of virtues are interrelated so that excellence of character and intelligence cannot be separated (cf. MacIntyre 2007: 154). Practice is historically embedded in following traditions, but is also open to change due to new understandings and values, thus through the exercise or lack of exercise of certain virtues (cf. ibid.: 222 f.).
[188] Cf. Elliott 1998: 38 f.
[189] Vieth 2010: 13.
[190] Cf Kirsh / Maglio 1994.
[191] Radoilska 2010: 370.

lectual achievement in its own right.[192] Radoilska proposes a theory of action that requires all of the following four forms of involvement in order to count as an agent's action: 1) the action is caused by an agent and 2) is attributable to an agent, 3) the agent is also responsible for the action or has feasible agential control over the action[193], and 4) the action is credible, i.e. the agent's commitment is expressed by the realization of some of the agent's values.[194] According to this definition, two actions could have the same outer effects, but differ »intrinsically« in nature and value. Besides, as an expression of agential control, an action is inherently valuable. Radoilska thus argues that an action that is brought forward with the help of enhancement methods both »devalues and downgrades« the action[195] such that »it cannot qualify as action proper, or praxis, which is also worthy independently from its desirable effects.«[196] If we would only consider the outer effects of an action without the intentions or thought processes that mirror the underlying values and virtues of the agent, epistemic harm is caused according to Radoilska. Because epistemic harm is instigated by the failure to appreciate intellectual achievement, the notion of cognitive enhancement, for Radoilska, implies a »Spartan-disposition« or »Spartan-like attitude to cognition«.[197]

Changing the cognitive phenomenology
A different but similar argument has been brought forth by Philip Walsh, who claims that enhancement is considered dangerous for our practice because it changes the »natural human cognitive phenomenology«, its »what-is-it-likeness«[198], which puts intellectual virtues at risk: there are possible repercussions for cognitive phenomenology that are disregarded and could lead to a revaluation of thinking, and thus of the notions of rationality, epistemic credit, and some intellectual virtues such as self-reliance and understanding.[199] Similar to Radoilska, Walsh recognizes the influence on cognitive achievements which are forms of agential involvement.[200] However, Walsh specifically focuses on the influence on our intellectual virtues like the »nature of conscious inference,« in which »one

---

[192] Radoilska 2010: 370.
[193] For the difference between attributability, control and responsibility cf. Shoemaker 2011.
[194] Cf. Radoilska 2010: 371 ff.
[195] Ibid.: 373.
[196] Ibid.: 374.
[197] Ibid.: 374 f.
[198] Walsh 2017: 35.
[199] Cf. ibid.: 44.
[200] Cf. ibid.: 47; Radoilska 2010: 371 ff.

has a sense of natural meaning«[201], as expressed in self-reliance. When self-reliance is undermined, so is the cultivation of other cognitive skills and abilities that can then not be exercised properly which, in turn, undermines true understanding.[202] Walsh concludes that if we are to design and use »authentic cognitive enhancement« in any form, then we should not only seek »functional integration« but also »phenomenal integration.«[203] How this could be possible is a matter of further discussion.

The misconceptualization of human agency

Fabrice Jotterand identifies limits to a person's development of character and value in his virtue ethical approach. He focuses on the aretaic categories, i. e. categories pertaining to virtue or excellence, of empathy, solidarity, altruism, gratitude, justice/fairness, shame, and forgiveness. Jotterand aims at explaining why neural moral enhancement »does not capture the fullness of human moral psychology, which includes moral capacity (ability or disposition to respond morally) and moral content (particular beliefs, moral actions, and ideas).«[204] This is to say that both moral capacity and moral content are natural and valuable in their own right. Jotterand also emphasizes the Aristotelian concept of *phronēsis* as well as virtues that entail types of »habitus or disposition of character acquired by the practice of morally good deeds.«[205] In order to accomplish *phronēsis* and move to excellence, human beings need to engage in the process of learning and understanding, which includes the ability to accept and correct mistakes. In a similar, but more precise way than the accounts discussed before, Jotterand argues that enhancement influences our emotions to the extent that it is difficult to determine what levels of emotional control for moral behaviour are considered adequate and what degrees of empathy is needed: »Virtue is a behavioral habit under the supervision of reason that can be taught and learned. The control and manipulation of moral emotions by technological means reduce the human mind to neurochemical mechanistic processes and threaten the very essence of moral agency, that is autonomy.«[206] The crucial point in Jotterand's critique is the distinction between character traits that describe the way of carrying out activities and having a character, which describes »a person's moral strength to establish a set of behaviors deemed adequate in projected circumstances«

---

[201] Walsh 2017: 46.
[202] Cf. ibid.: 47.
[203] Ibid.: 48.
[204] Jotterand 2011: 3.
[205] Ibid.: 7.
[206] Ibid.

as well as »qualifies one's moral agency and presupposes one's capacity of self-determination«.[207] While agency covers reasons, motives, and intentions, action constitutes character traits which only then lead to having a certain character. However, because transhumanism misconceptualizes moral agency, it cannot generate a content-full moral framework that adequately conceptualizes the virtues. Instead, such a framework would result in a misbalance between moral feelings and moral reasoning as well as it would have to remain silent about the nature of individual or social morality. Jotterand concludes that since moral emotions and moral reasoning constitute two inseparable elements of moral judgement, »moral neuroenhancement is unlikely to morally enhance in the true meaning of the word.«[208]

Some commonalities
The virtue ethical arguments against enhancement discussed in the preceding sections include various versions of the argument of inauthenticity and employ different aspects of authenticity. In its general outline, the argument of inauthenticity is closely related to the argument of naturalness, according to which dispositions, traits, or competences are naturally given and should be valued as such. This valuable human nature includes autonomy, the praxis of moral judgement (Sandel, Elliot, and Vieth) as well as the development of practical wisdom and rationality (Jotterand). It depends on practicing and improving virtues like self-reliance (Walsh, Radoilska). The argument from naturalness relies on an alleged »natural demarcation« between human beings on the one side and artificial means or things on the other side. It is usually complemented with an argument according to which any intervention in the human body or human mind not only affects the »true given nature« of human beings, but distorts core competences as expressed in human practices. Particularly, it is argued that the manipulation of agency through enhancement leads, if it is feasible at all, to a weaker and imperfect formation of virtues which in turn results in an erosion of human character.

5.1.2.7 Hubris and playing god
Proponents of restrictive positions occasionally accuse proponents of enhancement of the desire of »playing god«. Moreover, they suggest that various kinds of enhancements can be considered as hubris. Note that those levelling this accusation can give it a non-religious form: instead of

---

[207] Jotterand 2011: 8.
[208] Ibid.

the original argument (»doing x is playing god and should therefore not be allowed«), they can replace »is playing god« by stating that carrying out the task in question reliably and justifiably requires a level of expertise, knowledge etc. which is not available to human agents (now or in principle). In this version, the argument does not suggest that there is in fact an entity, which can reliably and justifiably carry out the action in question. It does, however, carry the same evaluation and action guidance for human agents, namely that they do and will not meet the standards required by the action in question. Given this general reading, some of the arguments referring to a specific aspect of human nature as changed only by the act of hubris can be read along secular lines.[209] In particular, Sandel's argument from the givenness of human nature has been defended with this strategy. Opponents had repeatedly challenged Sandel's argument, stating that it presupposed the belief in a divine creator to whom one can be grateful for being given a nature.[210]

Nevertheless, most typically the argument is guided by theological assumptions and the idea that it is against God's will to alter nature in general (cf. Lustig 2008). This presupposes knowledge about God's will and how He* determines the place of humans in nature. According to some opponents of enhancement, a promising option might be found in the literature of the diverse religious traditions. For reasons of brevity, we will only shortly discuss the perspective of the Christian tradition. An overview of religious arguments on enhancements from other traditions can be found in a special issue of *The Journal of Law, Medicine & Ethics*.[211] The underlying thought might be best described as a hope that the appeal to scripture, tradition, or church authority can justify a certain model that restricts usages of enhancement. Proponents of enhancement gave several rejoinders: initially, some stressed the point that opponents of enhancement must be aware of the temptation that human authorities themselves face to »play god« in interpreting God's will. Thus, the danger is that they may fall victim to their own argument. Moreover, and even more striking, is the response that the common models discussed in the Christian literature are not obviously build to support a restrictive position. For instance, Tony Coady differentiates three main models for conceiving human's role in nature, namely domination, co-creation and stewardship.[212] The first model places human nature under human dominion, and so leaves no

---

[209] For human nature arguments cf. section 5.1.2.5 (»Human nature and its components«).
[210] Cf. Giubilini / Sanyal 2015.
[211] The Journal of Law, Medicine & Ethics 2008: 36/1.
[212] Cf. Coady 2009: 157–160.

foothold for the enhancement objector. The same applies to the second model which starts from the Fall of Man, and therefore interprets nature as constituently depraved. Accordingly, now the task of humans is to correct this misfortune by acting as co-creators or shapers of the natural order alongside God. The third model makes humans responsible for the stewardship or care of nature. Obviously, this model imposes more constraints on human actions, allowing to criticize actions that transgress God's will for humans in handling their own or others nature. Nonetheless, any plausible account of stewardship which does not intend to go back to hunting and gathering societies must allow that appropriate care extends beyond the conservation of the natural order. It includes at least some shaping of its surroundings and its own nature. This is not to say that enhancement must be a part of this shaping. However, even the stewardship model does not rule out enhancement either. It only carves out that it is still a debatable question in the camp of the supporters of Christian assumptions.

In conclusion, the task to support the ›playing god‹-argument by solely pointing to the Christian tradition is not as self-evident as one might think at first view. There are several interpretations of the models that describe the relation of humans to the natural order. On a closer investigation, none of them is an undisputable option for opponents of enhancement. They can equally be introduced as enhancement friendly. Therefore, an opponent of enhancement needs further reasons why his favoured model actually endorses his critical line of argument.

5.2 Enhancement in social interaction

The arguments examined so far considered enhancement from an individual's point of view. In contrast, the core question of this section is: does it matter to our everyday interaction with friends and strangers whether they use biotechnological enhancement? The dialogical situation plays a comparably small role in the debate about enhancement. Most contributions are concerned either with the effect of enhancement on individual welfare or on larger social structures.

Nevertheless, there are some contributions, which try to identify and evaluate possible effects of biotechnological enhancement on dialogical interaction or to scrutinize how such enhancement relates to common social norms of interaction. Among these, the counterarguments prevail, i. e. biotechnological enhancement is more often seen as a threat to close social interaction than as a chance.

5.2.1 Supporting arguments

5.2.1.1 *The emotional basis of social interaction*

Biotechnological means can be used to influence the emotional basis of intimate relationships, be it in order to support fidelity and pair bonding[213], or to reduce emotional attachment in abusive or otherwise problematic relationships.[214] While the second effect, the ability to get rid of harmful attachments, might be subsumed under individual benefits, the former option is thought to affect all participants in the relationship positively. The idea behind modifying the emotional basis of social interaction is to either to remove emotional obstacles to social interaction or to promote the ability to engage in such interaction where it is desired. Given that successful and fulfilling social interaction is a good, this is a prima facie moral reason for this type of enhancement.

While this might at first sound quite abstract, some authors tend to refer to a set of concrete examples of possible biotechnological interventions and discuss animal studies where the effects have been shown in principle. The core idea is to manage behaviour, in particular sexual behaviour, which has a major influence on human pair bonding. One method of doing so could be the increase of sexual desire in the presence of the partner using pheromones or testosterone and the decrease of desire in the absence of the partner by means of the relevant antagonists. Another method discussed by Savulescu and Sandberg targets attachment between partners by modifying the level of oxytocin, vasopressin and corticotropin-releasing hormones.[215] The research on which this latter method is based has been conducted with prairie voles, which could be manipulated into increased or lowered pair-bonding by modulating their oxytocin- and vasopressin levels.[216] This mechanism might even be available for non-sexual relationships.

5.2.2 Counterarguments

5.2.2.1 *Social disruption*

How would a human talk to a posthuman, i. e. a person so strongly enhanced that he or she possesses some cognitive or emotive capacity on a level not obtainable by a human being? Would the posthuman have to

---

[213] Cf. Savulescu / Sandberg 2008.
[214] Cf. Earp et al. 2013.
[215] The various neuroscientific interventions into human pair bonding are discussed in Savulescu / Sandberg 2008: 35 ff.
[216] Cf. e. g. Insel / Hulihan 1995; Cho et al. 1999.

dumb down his communication style in order for a conversation to be possible? And if so, would he able to do so? This is a question that has been examined by a number of writers, including Fritz Allhoff and colleagues[217] as well as Nick Bostrom.[218] Bostrom focuses on commitments a newly enhanced posthuman might have or retain towards his unenhanced partner rather than on the communicative situation. The whole scenario presupposes that posthumans have radically different preferences, needs and abilities than humans. Bostrom presents the case of Mr. Bloggs, who becomes a posthuman by means of biotechnological interventions, and his wife Mrs. Bloggs. Bostrom wonders whether given the relationship with Mrs. Bloggs and their joint projects, this change might be bad for Mr. Bloggs. He argues as follows: Mr. Bloggs has a commitment not to contravene Mrs. Bloggs' preferences and she has a preference for him not to become posthuman. Given that it is bad for humans to forfeit their commitments, it might thus be bad for Mr. Bloggs to become posthuman.[219] This is, however, not the only way to look at the case of the Bloggs. Bostrom's argument can be made stronger than it is in his original presentation.

One does not have to assume these very specific preferences and commitments for Mr. and Mrs. Bloggs. The case is probably more interesting —and more tragic—if these two merely have preferences to advance shared projects such as joint hobbies, designing and creating a shared home, raising children etc., which rely on both of them having similar or at least compatible needs and preferences. This particular basis of needs and preferences is what some authors see as endangered by biotechnological enhancements. Additionally, common needs and preferences are a necessary condition for shared projects. This last claim needs further examination than has yet been presented in the debate. One can distinguish three cases: a) Two or more people have comparable and compatible preferences and engage in realising some project which fulfils these preferences, b) two or more people have comparable but conflicting preferences and engage in a process of negotiation and subsequent realisation of the compromise, c) two or more people have incomparable but compatible preferences and engage in a project which promises to fulfil the preferences of one of them. While in case a) and b) it is reasonable to speak of a shared project, case c) seems to be of a different kind. Here some people help others in realising their preferences without being committed to this

---

[217] Cf. Allhoff et al. 2010: 21.
[218] Cf. Bostrom 2008.
[219] Ibid.: 126 f.

realisation itself. Even if those who help others are strongly invested in the well-being of the person whose preferences are being realised, this is not a shared project but some kind of support of an individual project. This scenario is the dramatic version of what Mr. and Mrs. Bloggs might have to face if he becomes a posthuman. While he is still deeply interested in Mrs. Bloggs' well-being, still works alongside her to realise her preferences, his actions have lost what made them part of a shared project. He merely supports a project that ceased to be his, for reasons of indirect preferences in the fulfilment of Mrs. Bloggs' direct preferences.

Allhoff and colleagues explicitly turn to the problems of communication across persons with different mental abilities. Referring to Ludwig Wittgenstein's example of the talking lion who would not be understood by humans because they do not have a shared lifeform, they point out that radical enhancement such as the acquisition of new sensory modalities might undermine the shared basis of communication.[220] Allhoff's argument can draw on the background of the embodied mind theory, which seems to demonstrate that the bodily structure of a species shapes its cognition.[221] Beings with a significantly different embodiment—such as Thomas Nagel's famous bat[222]—are sure to have different ways of conceiving of, structuring, and communicating about their environment. It is, however, quite unclear whether quantitative changes in cognitive abilities might result in a similar kind of communicative gap as qualitative changes, such as different embodiments. Even the differences in cognitive structure brought about by differences in embodiment will vary significantly. As Allhoff and colleagues point out, serious differences in perceptive ability, i. e. blindness and sightedness, do not create a serious communication gap.[223]

5.2.2.2   *Coercion to enhance and rising standards*
Might the change in individual relations brought about by biotechnological enhancement of one partner result in unjustified negative consequences for the other(s)? As far as collective effects are concerned, the answer surely is affirmative. As will be discussed below, engaging in any kind of human enhancement will—amongst other effects—result in a change in the social standards for certain abilities, and this, in turn, will put pressure on the non-enhanced. But it is not clear whether negative

---

[220] Cf. Wittgenstein 1999: 223.
[221] For an overview cf. Shapiro 2011.
[222] Cf. Nagel 1974.
[223] A similar argument has been developed in Cabrera / Weckert 2012.

effects are limited to collective effects or can already occur in more limited cases of dialogical social interaction.

There are several cases in which the solitary user of biotechnological enhancement changes a social practice or event for everybody. The most obvious example is sports. The moral issues of doping do not only emerge once several participants dope and the norms for athletic performance rise. It is already sufficient that one single individual with significantly enhanced abilities participates.[224] As Thomas Douglas argues, the results of athletic competition would change depending on the willingness to engage in biotechnological intervention in addition to the current factors.[225] While there is nothing inherently problematic in a person's willingness to engage in biotechnological enhancement, its inclusion in sports and other competitive practices implies a considerable change in the practice in question, one which other participants might have good reasons to reject.

This argument has repeatedly been countered for the case of sports by pointing out that the use of biotechnological interventions can even mitigate another form of unfairness, namely the influence of the genetic lottery and social background. Enhancement technologies are often cheaper than advanced training gear and thus allow athletes from poorer countries to perform on the same level. Genetic background is morally arbitrary and allowing it to influence the outcome of the competition can be considered unfair.[226] While both arguments are valid, they need to be balanced against the one from changing the practice against possible good reasons of participants who intend to participate in a competition without being enhanced. What Douglas and others need to show is not that the competitive practice in question is fairer without the use of enhancement. They merely have to insist that some participants have good reason not to engage in biotechnological enhancement within the practice in question. The moral issue, then, is neither one of fairness nor one of breaking rules of a given practice. The issue is one of coercing others to change a practice they engage in.

---

[224] This might not be specific to biotechnologically enhanced capacities. The participation of exceptionally gifted athletes already changes the contest for everybody, including that athlete.
[225] Cf. Douglas 2015.
[226] Cf. Savulescu et al. 2004; Foddy / Savulescu 2007; Kayser et al. 2007.

5.2.2.3   *Complicity and its consequences*

One of the oldest arguments in the debate about human enhancement is the ›complicity‹-argument. In its generic form, the complicity argument claims that by engaging in some particular form of human enhancement, the user or an advisor or doctor can become complicit in establishing and promoting problematic social norms.[227] By using skin lightener or by cosmetic surgery transforming a hooked nose into an aquiline nose, one might become complicit with racial stereotypes; by using botox, filler, or liposuction, one might become complicit with sexist stereotypes or body ideals.

The argument can be developed in different ethical frameworks, namely in a consequentialist or deontologist version. In this section, we focus on the consequentialist interpretation of the argument.[228] On this reading, the argument draws attention to the *negative consequences* of complicity, i.e. that one in fact endorses a social norm and facilitates the negative effects of this norm on those who do not conform with it. Thus, collective harm—stabilizing problematic social norms—goes hand in hand with individual harm to those who do not undergo the enhancement procedure in question.[229] There is, however, an additional dimension to the argument which calls for discussing it under the current heading ›enhancement in social interaction‹. As the term ›complicity‹ already indicates, the idea is that the advisor or doctor takes part in a morally problematic practice, thus supports moral misdemeanour on the side of his patient or customer. While this does not necessarily make the doctor or advisor responsible for the consequences of the misdemeanour, it seems to be at odds with his or her vocation. This version of the argument depends on whether the social norm in question is indeed morally blameworthy and whether it results in real harm. For many social norms which seem to call for human performance enhancement, such as an achievement orientation of society, this has not been shown sufficiently.

5.2.2.4   *Complicity and its intrinsic badness*

Sometimes, complicity arguments are not brought forward in a consequentialist fashion, but in deontological terms. Traditionally, the deontological strand of the argument was designed and put forward in the context of cosmetic surgery. There, Margaret O. Little argues that cosmetic surgery to alter one's appearance might be consciously or subconsciously

---

[227] For a critical analysis cf. Ravelingien et al. 2009.
[228] For its deontological counterpart cf. section 5.2.2.4 (»Complicity and its intrinsic badness«).
[229] Cf. Boldt / Maio 2009.

in conspiracy with the suspect social norm of beauty, insofar as that surgery endorses the norm.[230] Note that this argument is not understood along consequentialist lines. The point is not that the compliance with an unjust norm *causes or leads to* certain consequences (e.g. unjust policy, society or culture). Rather, the wrong-making feature is the pure participation in a debatable practice guided by morally suspect norms. Little's negative example is an African-American who wants to look whiter. A doctor who offers treatment or the patient who strives for this kind of enhancement is complicit with norms that reflect or reinforce an unjust practice, in this case racism.

While complicity plays an important role in ethical debates about cosmetic surgery, there is less literature in the case of psychopharmacology. One reason for this might be that there is less agreement on the injustice of the norm. Of course, some may think of society's appreciation of cognitive performance, 24/7 economic activity, or continuous cheerfulness as undesirable and resist the pursuit of these by way of psychopharmacology. However, it would be difficult to argue that these norms are immoral and that certain enhancements make you an accomplice to an unjust practice. In this respect, there seems to be a difference between the norms that underlie cosmetic surgery and neuropharmacological interventions.[231] Therefore, restrictive positions need other reasons that can question pharmacological interventions. Elliott claims, for instance, that the current focus of society on competition leads not only to more productivity and economic wealth, but also to consequences like social coercion, loss of individuality, depression and feelings of inferiority.[232] Thus, by prescribing certain drugs, doctors support people to adapt to the questionable consequences of the competitive rat race. A case in point is the prescription of Modafinil to shift workers in order to get rid of their sleep disorders. Although the doctors might have good intentions, they can also be seen as complicit with the demands of society for high-performing workers and endorse direct or indirect forms of coercion.[233]

There are several critical replies that have been explored against the complicity argument, most of them well-known from previous debates in medical ethics.[234] To start with, the argument can be criticized for not being very precise about the different aspects of complicity. For instance,

---

[230] Cf. Little 1998.
[231] For this point cf. Schermer et al. 2009: 83.
[232] Cf. Elliott 2003.
[233] Cf. Appel 2008.
[234] Cf. e.g. Friele 2000.

there are many context factors (e. g. timing, proximity, certitude, knowledge, and intention) which are relevant to assess the normative force of the charge.[235] An overall evaluation must take these context factors into account, otherwise it falls victim to overgeneralization. Moreover, one might also question the dystopian analysis on which the argument relies: is a competitive practice in fact a morally corrupt social norm as the proponent of the complicity argument claims? And if so, why is this social norm corrupt, other than that it might have negative consequences? Here the complicity argument must join the dots between the practice and its negative moral status without falling back on purely consequentialist thinking. This means that one must show that the practice is unethical in a way that justifies the use of the concept of complicity in the first place. Moreover, some have stressed that the complicity argument relies on a biased weighing of unjust or unethical norms. This is because it seems still an open question whether moral corruption of a competitive practice does in fact outweigh the benefits of enhancement. In contrast, some have even argued for the opposite, namely that the opportunity costs of not enhancing are higher than the anticipated social pathologies or injustice.[236]

5.2.2.5 _Cheating_

One frequently used argument in the discussion about human enhancement is that the latter is or involves an act of cheating. As many other arguments against the use of enhancement, this argument has been originally suggested by the President's Council on Bioethics in its 2003 report. In general, the cheating accusation is well-known in the context of doping in sports. However, the Council has also used it with regard to cognitive enhancement in the context of education, exams, and the job market. The main rationale for the cheating argument refers to the implicit or explicit violation of the rules of the praxis in question.

MacIntyre's already introduced discussion of practices and their inherent rules, virtues, and goals[237] is the original inspiration of this argument.[238] According to MacIntyre, the goals of a practice such as sports cannot be realized without conforming to the practice-inherent rules and developing specific virtues.[239] There are different possible rules men-

---

[235] Cf. Orr 2007: 23.
[236] Cf. e. g. Levy 2013.
[237] Cf. section 5.1.2.6 (»Limits to the development of character and virtue«), subsection _The burden of responsibility._
[238] Cf. MacIntyre 2007.
[239] The argument from cheating has also been developed in a virtue ethical fashion which

tioned in the literature that enhancers are said to violate. According to Eric Juengst, for example, the use of Ritalin would undermine the disciplined study and active learning that the practice of being a student is supposed to involve.[240] Proponents of a permissive stance on enhancement have quickly noted that rules of competition can be unjustified in the first place so that a violation of such rules might be morally acceptable or even obligatory. Viewed in this light, the cheating argument against enhancement is conditional in nature.[241] Other proponents have pointed out that even if specific rules are justified, there need not be any violation by enhancers.[242] However, it might be said that these critical reactions are too dismissive of the value of such rules. There might be basic rules to different practices that are worth taking more seriously. For instance, one widely shared intuition is that success in a competition should depend on one's own merit rather than on drugs that enhance cognitive performance. Stephen Rose expresses this common intuition by saying that the use of steroids by athletes »at least in a competitive context, is seen as a form of cheating, of bypassing the use for hard work and study.«[243] And Michael Gazzaniga asks:

>»Why do we resist changes in our cognitive skills through drugs? It seems to me that it is because we think cognitive enhancement is cheating. If, somehow, someone gets better through hard work, that's okay. [...] But popping a pill and mastering the information after having read it only once seems like cheating.«[244]

This line of thought faces several challenges. First, it might be questioned whether the justification on the basis of merit is philosophically viable for deontologists. The reason for this is that merit is traditionally identified as a normative characteristic of the person and not the action itself. Therefore, the argument could fit better in the framework of virtue ethics in which personal characteristics have their natural habitat. Second, even if one ignores this classification issue, it is worth pointing out that the merit objection shows that enhancement is wrong independently of whether it is an act of cheating or not. It is not the pure act of cheating that makes enhancement wrong. The wrongness of any action, including enhance-

---

highlights the negative influence on character and therefore on the individual good life. Cf. for example Chatterjee 2004. For virtue ethical arguments cf. also section 5.1.1.3 (»Support of character and virtue development«) and section 5.1.2.6 (»Limits to the development of character and virtues«).

[240] Cf. Juengst 1998: 29–47.
[241] Cf. Savulescu et al. 2004.
[242] Cf. Ach et al. 2018.
[243] Rose 2005: 303.
[244] Gazzaniga 2005: 73.

ment, depends on the rules given by the spirit of the activity that include the relevant characteristic of merit.[245] Seen from this perspective, the crucial question is not whether enhancement is an act of cheating or not, but which normative constraints a certain activity should include and which not. If, for example, it turned out that the normative constraints imposed on athletes in sports are morally unfounded, violations of these rules would not be a wrong-making characteristic of enhancement *per se*. Evaluating the normative constraints of a given practice might be a difficult task in itself, especially within the realms of education and the job market.[246] More importantly, however, it leads us away from the straightforward notion of cheating-as-rule-breaking, into discussions on the rules, ends and goods of a certain activity that cheating is a part of.

5.3 Enhancement in social policy

Several arguments addressing the social effects of biotechnological enhancement presuppose that it is to be weighed according to its effect on fair social competition. And while competition is one of the main means of organising social cooperation, this widely shared presupposition of the competitive model of social cooperation strongly influences the subsequent argumentation. A majority of arguments aimed at social policy have envisioned scenarios about the future development of our principal models of cooperation. While there is significant leeway in the process of designing such scenarios, several developments have featured in many versions, amongst them the hope for social utility generated by the enhanced and the threat of diverse forms of social coercion and polarisations of society.

Beyond the mere exchange of arguments for and against the use of biotechnological interventions, the debate about human enhancement has resulted in a number of policy suggestions. Such suggestions have been developed for enhancement in general and for specific methods of enhancement in particular. Here, we can only provide examples for such regulatory suggestions, because this part of the debate has quickly started to thread into the specifics of medical regulations, drug regulations, social policy and many areas of specialised regulatory discourse.

One far-reaching regulatory framework has been proposed by Buchanan, who suggests an international organisation in charge of the licensing

---

[245] Cf. Giubilini / Sanyal 2015.
[246] Cf. Schermer 2008.

of innovations which are suited for human performance enhancement. The goal pursued by installing such an institution would be to solve what Buchanan calls *the diffusion problem*, i.e. the problem that some innovations do not reach poorer populations fast enough to prevent extreme deprivation or new economic and political inequalities.[247]

A fairly specialised regulatory framework can be found in the work of Hannah Maslen, who has based her contribution on the model of medical law. Her framework was particularly aimed at non-invasive neurostimulation devices such as Transcranial Magnetic Stimulation (TMS) and transcranial Direct Current Stimulation (tDCS).[248] She suggested to include enhancement technologies in an expanded medical devices regulation. Maslen modified her original (2014) framework later-on in cooperation with other prominent authors.[249]

In the following, we will not go any deeper into the discussion of regulatory frameworks, which we think should be left to experts in the legal field. Instead, we focus on the ethical arguments for and against the use and dissemination of means for human enhancement as far as its role in larger society is concerned.

5.3.1 Supporting arguments

5.3.1.1 *Mitigation of global catastrophic risks*
Global catastrophic risks[250] or ultimate harms[251] are events which will destroy or make inaccessible everything of value, e.g. end human civilisation, or make the planet uninhabitable. The possibility of such events has inspired several philosophical investigations. Before the obvious practical question of how to prevent or mitigate such an event can be tackled, intricate epistemological and practical questions have to be addressed, including ›What is the exact risk of such an event?‹ and ›How many resources are to be spend on estimating this risk?‹ While most attention has been spent on questions of epistemology and risk assessment[252], this kind of event has sparked interest in the enhancement debate as well. Might it be possible to enable human beings to predict, prevent, or miti-

---

[247] Cf. Buchanan 2011b: chapter 8.
[248] For ethical debates about transcranial stimulation cf. Illes / Gallo / Kirschen 2006; Heinrichs 2012.
[249] Maslen et al. 2015.
[250] Cf. Bostrom / Cirkovic 2008.
[251] Cf. Persson / Savulescu 2012.
[252] Cf. e.g. Munthe 2019.

gate extinction events and global catastrophic risks by biotechnological means? That this might be the case has been a thesis brought forward in discussions about the risk of unfriendly AI.[253] On the other hand, improved cognitive power combined with unchanged competitive tendencies stands a good chance to increase, not reduce, the risk of ultimate harm.[254] What keeps some people from understanding or at least from conceding an existential risk are not cognitive, but rather motivational factors as can also be seen in the debate on climate change.

Because cognitive improvement without moral changes will result in or at least not mitigate global catastrophic risks, Ingmar Persson and Savulescu have presented the idea of using moral enhancement for this task in a number of contributions. In a nutshell, their argument is this: Cognitive enhancement increases the number of people who can cause great harm, be it maliciously or negligently. Via promoting scientific progress, cognitive enhancement also increases the sheer amount of harm an individual can do. The probability that any individual realises her or his potential to do harm stays equal. Thus, cognitive enhancement increases the risk of harm and ultimate harm in the world. The only available and politically justifiable way of reducing this harm is by reducing the probability that individuals realise their potential to cause harm. This is most efficiently done by moral enhancement.[255]

This position has been attacked by a number of authors, but rarely because critics found it empirically implausible that moral enhancement might reduce the probability of harm, but rather because of the moral and political costs of this endeavour.[256]

5.3.1.2   Creation of social value

A famous argument by John Rawls justifies certain forms of inequality. Advantages of some are justified by the increase in welfare they generate for others. This argument targets primarily the entrepreneurial group, who, according to Rawls, should profit from their activities depending on the social value they generate.

»The inequality in expectation is permissible only if lowering it would make the working class even more worse off. [...] the greater expectations allowed to entrepreneurs encourages them to do things which raise the long- term prospects of the

---

[253] Cf. Yudkowsky 2008.
[254] Cf. Phoenix / Treder 2008: 494.
[255] Cf. Persson / Savulescu 2008; id. 2012; id. 2014.
[256] For a discussion on the critics cf. Harris 2011; Sparrow 2014.

laboring class. Their better prospects act as incentives so that the economic process is more efficient, innovation proceeds at a faster pace, and so on.«[257]

The same argument has been employed for users of biotechnological enhancement. If human enhancement were to enable some individuals to generate more social value than they could otherwise provide, this would count as a reason for a permissive stance towards enhancement, or even for some supportive social mechanisms: »Enhancements for a few that enable them to better solve the world's environmental problems would satisfy Rawls' difference principle in that the extra inequality in ability would help the worst off.«[258]

In a similar vein, Buchanan argues that biotechnological enhancements should be regulated so that social value is increased. Just as other innovations, biotechnological enhancement can even generate social value if it is not (yet) universally available. Buchanan compares biotechnological enhancement to non-biotechnological forms, such as literacy: Even though the latter was initially a privilege of a rich elite, it provided social value for the whole of society, which benefited from the communicative and administrative services made possible by this elite.[259] Enhancement often is a positive-sum event for society.

5.3.1.3 _Creation of equality of chances_
Biotechnological enhancement might not only be used in order to generate extreme abilities so as to counter risks currently not open to human mitigation, or to generate social value beyond what is feasible today. It has also been claimed that it can be used to decrease inequalities, by enhancing those with lesser talents and abilities.

Early Rawls-inspired contributions to the enhancement debate argued that a just medical system provides therapeutic interventions only. This claim was supported by pointing out that therapy is suited to enable everybody to contribute to social cooperation according to his given talents. Enhancement, in contrast, was considered to lie beyond the limits of such a just medical system.[260] This suggestion was rather restrictive as far as the role of human enhancement is concerned. Enhancement was considered to be a means towards ends, which other members of the society had no reasons to contribute to. Thus, it did not belong to a social support system—health care—which supported all members of society in

---

[257] Rawls 1971: 78.
[258] Allhoff et al. 2010: 18.
[259] Cf. Buchanan 2011a: 110.
[260] Cf. Daniels / Sabin 1997.

reaching aims, which others do have reasons to contribute to, namely, to take part in social cooperation.

Contrary to this rather restrictive position, later contributions suggest that biotechnological enhancement might not only generate new choices, but that it might thereby create more equality of chances.[261] The aim is, however, not to install genetic equality, but to strive for what the authors call a »decent genetic minimum«.[262] Nevertheless, the ideal of levelling the playing field, i. e. an integration of the natural lottery into distributional policies seems to linger in the seminal *From chance to choice* and Buchanan's later work. While he defends using biotechnological intervention even if it is not yet universally available, this universal availability remains the long-term objective.[263] Insofar as biotechnological enhancement ought to be *universally* available, equality is a goal, but insofar as it should only be universally *available*, the goal is not simply equality but equality of chances.

5.3.2 Counterarguments

Using enhancement might promise social benefits, but it also carries the threat of social disruptions. Such social disruptions can have various forms. Yet, they can be divided into three groups. The first group of negative effects on social life concerns the effects which the enhancement of some has on the cooperation and competition with those who do not undergo enhancement. The threats to social life, which fall under this category, are often some form of pressure on the unenhanced. The second group of threats affects the social cohesion of a society in which enhancement might change the composition of social groups. The last set of disruptions might affect the minimal social consensus about what counts as good in an individual life and in society.

5.3.2.1 *Discrimination of the enhanced / unenhanced*

Tensions and forms of discrimination between groups or individuals who perceive themselves to be part of some group are a sad constant of human history. It is not unlikely that the use of biomedical enhancement might be perceived as a criterion of group membership and thus a reason for differential treatment. This likelihood will vary with the specific type of enhancement, being quite high for more obvious and more permanent

---

[261] Buchanan et al. 2001.
[262] Ibid.: 82.
[263] Cf. Buchanan 2011a: 111 f.

enhancements—genetic enhancement in particular—and less likely for hidden, occasional enhancement such as the use of Ritalin for an exam.[264] Scenarios in which there are more or less identifiable groups of enhanced and unenhanced humans have been developed in science fiction as well as in serious philosophical writing. Differential treatment of unenhanced or enhanced persons might already result from simple ingroup-outgroup distinctions, but there are more complex reasons, which have been discussed in ethical literature.

One of the most impressive scenarios has been depicted by Daniel Wikler.[265] As in his previous work about paternalism towards people with lesser cognitive abilities[266], he points out that social standards are being developed with the conflicting aims of inclusion and efficiency. A social standard that allows for more efficiency, such as higher steps of stairs, will fail to include people with lower abilities in the relevant realm, in this case people with lower mobility. While standards can be devised to be more inclusive, they will nearly always exclude some persons for the sake of efficiency. This type of exclusion will often be carried out by a majority or by those who have some dominance in the discourse about social norms. Even a minority can—say by overrepresentation in digital media and the data collected in these media—shape such social norms and standards. Being excluded by social norms and standards is one relevant kind of discriminatory treatment. If social standards and norms are for some reason set by people who undergo biotechnological enhancement, it is quite likely that persons of average ability, or at least of what today counts as average ability, will be excluded by such norms. As mentioned, this need not occur because the enhanced are a majority; overrepresentation in the data or discourse through which norms are set can be sufficient.

The scenario developed by Lee Silver uses much less in-depth analysis of the social mechanisms that bring about social norms and standards.[267] Nevertheless, he tries to depict the development of a heavily polarized society, which has evolved from individual decisions, such as choice of partners, prevention of negative hereditary traits where possible, and some forms of genetic immunization, to a society standing at the brink of speciation. The decisive premise in Silver's scenario, which has later

---

[264] In- and outgroup effects have, however, been observed even for these less obvious cases of enhancement. Cf. for example the reports of collective studying behaviour, in which non-users were perceived as markedly different from the rest of the students in Wagner 2017.

[265] Cf. Wikler 2010.

[266] Cf. Wikler 1979.

[267] Cf. Silver 1997.

been explicitly called out as problematic by Buchanan, is that most of the individually chosen measures are to be paid for privately and are not supported by some social welfare mechanisms. Given this premise, Silver takes it to be highly probable that financial wealth gets transformed into biological wealth, which is why he calls the new genetically enhanced group »GenRich« which seems to be the shortcut for »genetically enriched« at first sight.

In Silver's scenario, it takes a couple of centuries to establish a fully polarized society, but once genetic manipulation and selection over generations has taken its course, the unenhanced, or ›Naturals‹, get disadvantaged in education and the job market. Silver explicitly claims that such persons would only receive minimal schooling, much below today's standards, and thus below what would be needed to let unenhanced people develop to their full potential. The job market would see the same form of segregation, giving all high responsibility jobs to the GenRich and leaving only simple work to the Naturals. Even if Silver concedes that there is a relevant distinction in ability, he does not assume that Naturals are not capable of carrying out more ambitious jobs. They are simple excluded from them.

5.3.2.2 _Coercion to enhance and rising standards_

The scenarios introduced by Wikler and Silver in which social norms and standards might rise due to the influence of people using biotechnological enhancement do not merely depict possible sources of discrimination.[268] They also contain one of the most plausible reasons why people unwilling to engage in biotechnological enhancement might come under pressure or even be coerced to do so anyway. Rising social standards can have such an effect in two different ways. On the one hand, there will simply be competition for social goods, in which biotechnological enhancement provides an advantage. The pressure to compete on a similar level can turn into pressure to engage in biotechnological enhancement, if the latter is a necessary or simply the most accessible path to equal chances in the competition.[269] This effect will only occur where social cooperation is organised as competition.[270] To be sure, several areas of social life are organised differently and will thus not provide an incentive to enhance. Nevertheless, in these areas another mechanism might have

---

[268] Silver 1997; cf. Wikler 2010.
[269] Cf. e. g. Farah et al. 2004; Sturma 2019: 142 f.
[270] For an argument that these areas of social life increase, cf. Galert et al. 2009.

similar effects, namely the enforcement of rising standards in social inter-action.

Rising standards and other norms requiring individuals to be en-hanced will most likely come to be enforced in a plethora of ways. One obvious—and maybe easier to mitigate—enforcement is active, institu-tional enforcement, ranging from employment policies of private compa-nies to criteria for welfare support by the state and plain and simple legal requirements. Less obvious, there is enforcement of norms and standards in social interaction, which can affect such diverse areas of conduct and ability as moral praiseworthiness[271], etiquette, cognitive or physical per-formance. If standards of moral praiseworthiness were to change in a way which excludes morally unenhanced individuals from ever being praised for moral conduct, this would probably provide some incentive to engage in biotechnological enhancement. Such a change could occur, for example, if mere morally allowed behaviour was socially taken for granted and only exceptional and supererogatory action received praise. The moral issue with rising standards is primarily that people not willing to engage in enhancement will be excluded from equal social participation. This seems to be a harm to these individuals even if society decided to install some protective institutional and legal measures to prevent economic harm or harm in legal standing.

A special version of the rising standards argument has been suggested by Dan Brock who coined the term »self-defeating enhancements«.[272] If the benefits of enhancement were purely positional and enough people gave in to the coercion to enhance, the effects would be self-defeating. Everybody would have to struggle harder just to stay in the same (socio-economic) place.

5.3.2.3   Enhancement divide

The idea of a divide of society or even mankind into the enhanced and the unenhanced has been presented in various versions by several authors. However, a general distinction should be made when talking about such a divide, namely whether it runs between humans and post-humans (Bostrom) or between persons and post-persons (Nicholas Agar), or both. The divide between humans and post-humans is predominantly biological, generated by alterations in the genetic structure of a part of humanity. It will be discussed below under the heading ›division of the

---

[271] Cf. Archer 2016.
[272] Brock 1998: 60.

species‹. The divide between persons and post-persons is predominantly concerned with abilities and needs, where post-persons are usually thought to have significantly higher abilities and possibly other and more extensive needs. These two divides can go hand in hand but need not. They are predominantly concerned with the differences in moral status and epistemic and cognitive abilities of individuals.

What came originally to be known as the enhancement divide is mainly a socio-economic divide, as has been demonstrated early on in Silver's and Wikler's scenarios alike. It is a form of social polarisation, typically along the line of wealth and access to enhancement technologies. The enhancement divide has its real-world predecessor in the so-called *digital divide*, the divide between persons who do have access to digital media, and in particular to internet services, and those who do not. Access to digital media generates social and economic opportunities not otherwise available and, as a consequence, has the potential to generate new inequalities or deepen existing ones. The concept of a digital divide has been contested and the empirical phenomenon so described has shifted from a divide in access to a divide in the type of interaction.[273] Nevertheless, it seems to be a good model for a possible enhancement divide, insofar as sociodemographic factors such as age, wealth, and education led to different access to a modern technology, which in turn led to different socioeconomic chances and status.

A similar development might well occur for biotechnological enhancement insofar as it is more accessible given a certain wealth and can be used safely only given a certain educational background. Biotechnological enhancement requires a fairly knowledgeable user. In order to enhance oneself successfully, one does have to know which cognitive process to target, which substance is suitable for this purpose, how to dose and how to identify and mitigate adverse effects, which pharmacological interactions to avoid, how long to use the substance, etc. Again, sociodemographic background has a strong influence on one's access to the technology, and the technology might have a strong influence on one's life chances.

Whether the probability of a socio-economic divide is a good reason against policies allowing or supporting enhancement depends on a number of factors, such as the value assigned to equality and the confidence in trickle-down effects. If, on the one hand, one assigns equality a separate, high value, a possible gain in overall welfare will not balance out the loss of equality. If, on the other hand, one values equality low or even assigns a

---

[273] Cf. Guillén / Suárez 2005.

mere derivative value to it, overall welfare gain will suffice to accept an enhancement divide.[274]

5.3.2.4 *Lack of social fit, supremacy and discrimination*
The previous scenarios share the assumption that people using biotechnological enhancement and those abstaining are cooperating and competing within a single social framework, if unequally and often antagonistically. An even more radical scenario might question whether a single social framework can be suitable to house the enhanced and the unenhanced alike. Radical enhancement, in particular, might have the potential to change the preferences and needs, the mode of communication of people so radically, that they are thoroughly estranged from institutions and regulations providing for the preferences and needs of the unenhanced.

The scenarios for such an extreme divide have rarely been developed outside science fiction literature. The closest candidates in academic writing probably are depictions of a so-called *mind-uploading*, i. e. the process in which the normal biological realization of the cognitive states and processes of a human person is replaced by a technical realization, or to oversimplify a bit: the transfer of mental states and processes from a human brain to some other computational machine.[275]

Uploading, according to a thesis from the transhumanist side, is only possible if functionalism is true.[276] Daniel Dennett points out that uploading considerations only make sense if a person's cognitive processes can be explained by patterns in the matter of the human body.[277] This means, in a nutshell, the fact that a state is present in a *biological* brain must not be decisive for the fact that it is a mental state. If mental states were not individuated by such a pattern but by their biological basis, as e. g. John Searle claims[278], then they could not be realized in another medium.

Some futurologists try to extrapolate possible technologies that can be used to replicate the consciousness of a human person in a technical medium. Current proposals differentiate between variants of this process that have different speeds, different structures, and different ways of dealing with the original. Without going into the concrete technological proposals here, Chalmers distinguishes between gradual and instantaneous

---

[274] Cf. e. g. Buchanan 2011a.
[275] Cf. Kurzweil 2005.
[276] Cf. More 2013: 6.
[277] Cf. Dennett 2012: 88 f.
[278] Cf. Searle 1980: 424.

forms. Both can be either destructive or sustaining.[279] Many authors believe that gradual uploading is the more promising candidate for maintaining a persistent person. The main reason for this is that the authors in question assume that every single replacement of the basis of realization preserves the realized consciousness unchanged. Given the current state of neuroscience and computational technology, uploading remains a rather remote possibility; we will therefore not go into any more technical details of the processes envisioned in the literature. Uploading is predominantly of interest here, because it can work as a showcase of how a single social framework for all humans and post-humans can become obsolete through radical enhancement. Uploaded post-humans and humans would probably not share enough in order to justify or even enable a shared culture, perhaps not even the temporal structure of thought and action.

5.3.2.5 Division of species

Another notion introduced by Silver is speciation by means of enhancement. The fact that biotechnological enhancement might result in the development of one or more new species is closely linked to genetic forms of enhancement. The suggestion is that two or more groups of humans across which sexual reproduction is impossible might develop due to biotechnological modification of the genome of some individuals and selective procreation amongst them. For the most part, non-genetic enhancement is not considered powerful enough for speciation except in science fictional literature. The scenario of speciation has been taken up from an ethical perspective[280] and within the philosophy of biology, in particular in the debate about the concept of human nature.[281] The latter shows that the term ›human nature‹ needs to be treated with more caution than sometimes found in the debate. The idea that enhancement technologies might either endanger human nature as a whole or endanger species membership for a few (as e.g. Fukuyama and Kass suggest) carries pre-Darwinian ideas of human nature, which are incompatible with modern biological science. Even the concept of human nature as used by Silver and Agar is not without alternative. Silver and Agar refer to the possibility of interbreeding as the criterion of species-membership and thus use a biological species concept. One common alternative is to refer to all members of an evolutionary lineage as the same species. Reproductive isola-

---

[279] Cf. Chalmers 2010: 33 ff.
[280] Cf. Agar 2007; Buchanan 2009a; id. 2011b.
[281] Cf. Lewens 2012.

tion of different subpopulations would not be a speciation event under this concept.[282]

A major part of the debate following Buchanan and Agar systematically refers to the divide between post-persons and persons, i.e. between individuals of strongly different ability sets and needs. Nevertheless, Agar refers to the divide as that between humans and post-humans while Buchanan distinguishes between the divides between humans and post-humans versus that between persons and post-persons. The core issues at hand for both is whether there might be beings with higher capabilities and whether more extensive needs might encourage them to claim a higher moral status than ordinary human beings.

Buchanan seems to doubt that such creatures are possible but admits that this might be due to a limitation of his own imagination. Even if such creatures should be possible, he denies that they would have a higher moral status. He admits, however, that there might be different sets of rights for different species. That would not be a limit or even a downgrading of human rights. Much to the contrary, Buchanan considers human rights as rights to the political, social and maybe material conditions of development. Such rights would gain in relevance and standing once their bearers enter into a disadvantageous relation to beings who might believe to have reason to limit or withhold such conditions of development.

Agar, on the other hand, suggests that it might be possible that post-humans have an even higher moral status than normal human persons and investigates what the consequences for the interaction between persons and post-persons might be.[283] One obvious effect has been observed by Jeff McMahan, who suggests that even inviolable moral status might come in grades and thus might allow for trade-offs.[284] If that were the case, the famous utilitarian trolley cases and their real-world counterparts of triage situations would be changed fundamentally. In case of the presence of post-persons, they would no longer generate moral dilemmas in which equal inviolable moral status has to be balanced against each other. Rather, they would allow for the comparison of the unequal moral status of different moral patients. Agar and Robert J. Sparrow devise similar scenarios and take it to be quite likely that post-persons will find reason to sacrifice mere persons for higher goals much as persons currently sa-

---

[282] Cf. Gyngell 2012.
[283] Cf. Agar 2013.
[284] Cf. McMahan 2009.

crifice non-personal but sentient beings.[285] As a consequence, both Agar and Sparrow warn against creating such beings of higher moral status.[286]

5.3.2.6   *Too much social homogeneity and lack of diversity*

A different radical scenario points out a possible development where access to enhancement is nearly universal and the aims which people pursue by biotechnological means are fairly similar. In this case, it is not to be expected that there will be an overabundance of social diversity. Quite the opposite, it might turn out that people become more and more alike at least in their capacities, the more they use the same enhancement technologies. Given that many enhancers work better for individuals on the lower end of the capacity spectrum for a given task and bring only little if any advantage for those already highly capable, this result is not unlikely.

That might become a burden for society too, because social cooperation is based on a distribution of labour according to the abilities and preferences of the participants. The division of labour is one of the strongest drivers of social cooperation and generates a major part of its surplus. Division of labour depends on a difference in talent and capability. It is not an arbitrary decision which part of the divided labour a person takes, but the decision is at least partly guided by that person's talents and preferences. If these talents and preferences are influenced by biotechnological intervention and happen to be modified towards more homogeneity, the division of labour can well become problematic. Moreover, the difference in talents and preferences plays a role in accounting for differences in hierarchical positions. The hierarchical structure of many current institutions might come under pressure from a homogenization via biotechnological means.[287]

A similar argument can be found in Chris Gyngell, who points out that cognitive diversity plays a major role in collective problem-solving capacity.[288] If there were some cognitive capacities to be perceived as general-purpose goods and pursued by means of biotechnological enhancement by a vast majority of individuals in society, this might reduce cognitive diversity with detrimental consequences for society.[289]

The idea that biotechnological enhancement might modify cognitive diversity has been modelled by game-theoretic means by Sandberg and

---

[285] Cf. Agar 2013; Sparrow 2013.
[286] The opposite conclusion, namely that we should create such beings, has been drawn by Rakic 2015 in a reply to Agar.
[287] Cf. Wasserman 2014.
[288] Cf. Gyngell 2012.
[289] Cf. ibid.: 508 f.

Joao Fabiano: because it is not possible to model the full diversity of talents and preferences within a society, they stuck to a variation in social value orientation, similar to a hawks-versus-doves-paradigm.[290] Their results lend some credibility to Wasserman's warning that social homogeneity might increase. They observed an increase in prosocial value orientation, if not a full removal of individuals with adversarial orientation.

5.3.2.7 Competition for social resources

Developing biotechnological enhancements requires time, effort, and material resources. These resources could be employed for other tasks such as the development of therapeutic technologies, support technologies, infrastructure etc. Thus, the development of biotechnological enhancement competes with other relevant social goals.[291] This competition takes place in a number of areas, e. g. in the research decisions of universities and corporations alike, in the decisions of public and private investors, in legislative procedures, in insurance policies etc. Given the number of decision processes in which this competition is played out, it is impossible to discuss all the diverse factions, interests and needs involved.

It has been doubted, in particular, whether the high-tech orientation dominating a major part of the enhancement debate is adequate. Focussing on high-tech interventions such as neurostimulation, psychopharmaceuticals or even brain-computer interfaces tends to obscure more simple interventions which can reach a larger part of the population. Laura Cabrera[292] has pointed out that a population health perspective is suited to draw attention away from individualistic, biotechnological interventions and towards interventions in psychological[293], social and technical infrastructure while still keeping the goal of enhancing human traits and performances in view. Given that low-tech interventions tend not only to be less resource-intensive, but also tend to affect a larger number of people, there are good reasons to socially invest in this type of enhancement rather than in supporting high-tech development.

This perspective might provide a counterargument to Buchanan, who makes the case that human enhancement technologies will most likely not (only) be a private market good, but subject to state-(re)-distribution and subsidy.[294] If it is indeed more effective to invest into low-tech interven-

---

[290] Cf. Sandberg / Fabiano 2017.

[291] Cf. Miah 2011.

[292] Cf. Cabrera 2015; id. 2017.

[293] Such a structure of nudges is discussed in Blumenthal-Barby / Burroughs 2012.

[294] Cf. Buchanan 2011a: 122 ff.

tions in order to enhance the capacities of a whole population, then state-investment into high-tech interventions becomes harder to justify and therefore rarer. If state investment in the form of substitutions, social enhancement-and-health care or similar solutions is rare and the state refrains from deterring measures such as taxes or prohibitions, it is quite likely that high-tech biotechnological enhancement will predominantly become a private market good.

A special case of competition for resources is perceived to take place between social and biotechnological solutions. A slightly dated example refers to the use of human growth hormone for instilling growth in smaller people instead of adjusting social infrastructure to suit people of different heights.[295] A more recent example discusses how concentration in classrooms can be facilitated either by using psychopharmacological enhancement or by simply reducing the size of classes.[296] These situations are special insofar as biotechnological enhancement in these cases is not intended to simply improve a person's capacities, but it is intended to enable people to conform to specific social norms. Enhancement is thus used to normalise people. A similar issue arises in the case of compensatory and therapeutic enhancements, where people with disabilities or uncommon abilities are confronted with the—usually well-meant—option to normalise their abilities via biotechnological interventions.[297] In the case of interventions with a clearly enhancing character, similar effects can occur, especially if social norms deviate significantly from people's abilities—a situation that can itself be caused or promoted by the spread of enhancement.[298]

5.3.2.8   Non-autonomous enhancement (military etc.)
Human performance enhancement is often pictured in scenarios which adhere to good biomedical practice, meaning that it is the user's desires that decide whether an intervention is undertaken or not. It is generally presupposed that user autonomy is protected by institutional processes such as informed consent procedures or enforceable consumer rights. This has been called liberal or autonomous in contrast to heteronomous enhancement. Obviously, this is not the only scenario for human performance enhancement. As a number of writers has pointed out, there are several possible scenarios in which hierarchies play an important role in

---

[295] Cf. Juengst 1998: 41f.
[296] Cf. Levy 2007. Cf. section 5.1.2.1 (»Adverse (and long-term) effects«).
[297] Cf. Silvers 1998.
[298] Cf. section 5.3.2.2 (»Coercion to enhance and rising standards«).

the decision about the use of a biotechnological enhancement. The most prominent scenario in this regard is that of military enhancement.[299] This scenario has a specific moral cast because membership in the military is in many cases not fully voluntary itself. Many nations draft young adults and sanction them—sometimes severely—for evading the draft. Compulsory biotechnological enhancement for draftees would thus run counter to the legitimatory practice of biotechnological interventions in general.

Military service is not the only possible constellation for not fully autonomous enhancement. There are draft systems beyond the military service in some countries, and in others the decision which career to pursue is strongly influenced by social, political, or even private hierarchies. The combination of such forced or strongly sanctioned choices and obligatory biotechnological enhancement regimes will result in similar borderline cases of justification.

The other type of enhancement, for which compulsory interventions have been suggested is moral enhancement.[300] In this particular case, the justification for biotechnological intervention is the prevention of ultimate harm.[301] Most authors take the biotechnological means for this task to be some form of genetic modification, amongst others because for some forms of pharmacological intervention it has been shown that its involuntary administration does not have the desired results.[302] Others have gone further and suggested that if one is to argue for compulsory moral bioenhancement, one should also argue for it to be conducted in covert programs.[303] Given that moral enhancement has significant conceptual and technical issues to solve before it is a viable option[304], compulsory solutions for it seem even more dubious.

5.3.2.9 _Changing an already optimal human nature_

Is the natural structure of human beings so complex that changes in one property will likely result in detrimental effects or even a collapse of the finely balanced whole? This is at least a risk pointed out by some participants in the debate, amongst others Kass and Fukuyama. If not extremely interconnected, the biological structure of human beings might be optimal or near optimal, given that it has developed across a long process of natural selection. Changes to this structure run the risk of substituting

---

[299] Cf. Mehlman et al. 2013; Lin et al. 2014.

[300] Cf. Persson / Savulescu 2008: 174. For counterarguments cf. Rakic 2014; Sparrow 2014.

[301] Cf. section 5.3.1.1 (»Mitigation of global catastrophic risks«).

[302] Cf. Rakic 2017.

[303] Cf. Crutchfield 2019.

[304] Cf. Beck 2015.

human tinkering for evolutionary craftsmanship.[305] This claim has been denounced by Buchanan in quite some detail, in particular by showing how it relies on a misconception of evolution as a master craftsman. He suggested replacing the metaphor of the master craftsmen or even the blind watchmaker by that of a morally blind, fickle, tightly shackled tinkerer.[306] What he wants to point out by this metaphor is that evolution does not serve human needs as a watchmaker does, nor does it treat human beings more or less equally. It does not have any foresight across current niches or evolutionary pressure, nor tools to make modifications across species rather than within a line of descendants.

6. Concluding observation

6.1 Summary: What is the enhancement debate all about?

From a distanced perspective, one could say that the enhancement debate is about the legitimate means of pursuing individual and collective benefits. When zooming in, the core question changes and becomes more fine-grained: are biotechnological enhancements a legitimate means of modifying the traits and abilities of individual humans and, if so, under which social and legal conditions?[307] This last question is helpful for structuring the different positions in the debate: some authors think that biotechnological enhancement is not a legitimate means to modify human traits and performances or only in rare cases. Examples for this point of view that have been examined in some detail in this expert report are the rationales of Sandel, Kass and the other members of the President's Council. They argue for restricting the use of technologies already existing and often vote for restricting their further development. They tend to concentrate on the counterarguments as presented above. Other authors do not merely think that biotechnological means are suited, but also that they are among the best means to an end which these authors endorse, namely human performance enhancement. This is a line of reasoning favoured for example by Harris, Bostrom, Persson and Savulescu. These authors tend to concentrate on the pro-arguments offered above. Finally,

---

[305] For an in-depth analysis of this line of reasoning cf. section 5.1.2.5 (»Human nature and its components«).

[306] Cf. Buchanan 2011a: 48f.

[307] A newer trend is to investigate if and how such conditions, once identified, can be brought about by concrete policy decisions or strategies, cf. section 5.3 (»Enhancement in social policy«).

there is a set of authors standing somewhere in the middle, accepting some of the pro- and some of the counterarguments and either opting for the individual's right to decide herself whether to use such means of self-modification or for policies targeting not enhancement in general, but specific interventions under specific circumstances for specific aims. Examples for this middle position are Buchanan, Judy Illes and Levy. Given the ripe state of the debate, it should not come as a surprise that almost every position feasible in the pro-contra-spectrum has been endorsed by some authors.

However, there are still some open paths in the debate and some theoretical impasses which are yet to circumnavigate. In the following, we want to make some suggestions.

6.2   What is the debate struggling with?

6.2.1   The placeholder-debates

The analysis shows that at least some arguments have the tendency for terminological gloss-over, which might lead away from the crucial ethical debate in question. This is true for many arguments, especially those that rely on the concepts of welfare[308], authenticity[309], naturalness[310], cheating[311] and complicity[312]. This is not to say that it is not possible to build a conclusive argument with these concepts. We are just pointing to the fact that if one tries to do so, one has to justify the *underlying rule, principle,* or *value* that is presupposed in the first place. Given that, we suggest that proponents of these arguments should put more emphasis on the justification of the real issues in question rather than on the characterisation of actions as—on the side of the permissive views—as welfare promoting and authentic or—on the side of the restrictive views—as unnatural, cheating or complicity. Interestingly, some arguments that refer to human nature seem to be more sensible to this challenge.[313] While the phrase ›against human nature‹ itself is vague and by far not self-explanatory as we have tried to show, there are different ways of making explicit what it is

---

[308] Cf. section 5.1.1.1 (»Improved welfare«).

[309] For arguments pro cf. section 5.1.1.2 (»Means of leading an authentic life«), for arguments against cf. section 5.1.2.4 (»Loss of authenticity«).

[310] Cf. section 5.1.2.5 (»Human nature and its components«) and section 5.1.2.6 (»Limits to the development of character and virtues«).

[311] Cf. section 5.2.2.5 (»Cheating«).

[312] Cf. section 5.2.2.4 (»Complicity and its intrinsic badness«).

[313] Cf. section 5.1.2.5 (»Human nature and its components«).

meant to refer to. They range from undermining a person's autonomy and dignity over threatening specific character traits to eroding a special relation to the universe. Therefore, the argument seems to make progress insofar as it clearly states what is at issue in the debate. However, whether any of these interpretations is justifiable is a highly debated question. This should not come as a surprise since arguments from human nature crisscross many enduring, broad topics and themes from diverse philosophical subdisciplines. Therefore, we support a broader philosophical discussion of this type of argument, including not only expertise from applied ethicists, but also from epistemology, philosophy of biology, and metaphysics.[314] The same suggestion can be made for arguments that refer to enhancement technologies as playing god or hubris.[315] In the case of understanding them in secular terms, they are solely placeholders for the ›real thing‹ that justifies the playing god accusation. At best, they are understood as variations of the human nature argument. In the case they are understood within a religious framework, it is far from self-evident that they can ground a challenge against enhancement not just because of their controversial metaphysics, but because even in the Christian tradition, the anti-enhancement interpretation is not without alternatives. In order to make progress, the theological dispute is in need for further justification, too.

6.2.2   The decisive reason assumption of the restrictive views

It is notable that some opponents of enhancement do not engage in a balancing of the pros and cons of legitimating enhancement. Rather, they lay out one or a few reasons against such a legitimation. For example, Sandel bases his case almost exclusively on the claim that engaging in enhancement expresses an objectionable attitude—an attitude of »mastery«.[316] He makes no attempt to weigh this concern against possible upsides of enhancement. This is a common, but by no means unquestionable strategy of most of the protagonists who favour a restrictive position. Why should the diagnosis that a technology is against human nature be a decisive reason against enhancement? This question is not raised very often in the debate, but we would like to flag it as one worth exploring

---

[314] Cf. for example the discussion of Lewens 2012 in the special issue »Evolution, Genetic Engineering and Human Enhancement« of the journal *Philosophy and Technology*.
[315] Cf. section 5.1.2.7 (»Hubris and playing god«).
[316] Cf. section 5.1.2.5 (»Human nature and its components«) and section 5.1.2.6 (»Limits to the development of character and virtues«).

further.[317] If one does, one also has to consider putting more thoughts into a solid theory that explains how to weigh the different arguments of the restrictive, permissive, or mandatory positions against each other.

6.2.3 The burden of proof strategy of the permissive views

As already stated above, many authors who favour permissive and mandatory views emphasize that there are good pro tanto reasons for enhancement, namely that it promotes the well-being of the agent.[318] But there is even more to that point. Several authors do also see reasons of welfare as a good dialectical move in order to shift the burden of proof. This shifts the evaluative default move as follows: enhancement is a good thing as long as there are no reasons that count against it. For instance, Buchanan states:

»Biomedical enhancements have provoked huge controversy. Given that enhancement isn't new and that it has played a central role in human progress, what's all the fuss? Why should we tie our hands, cut ourselves off from further progress, by forgoing enhancements just because they happen to use biomedical technologies?«[319]

In this passage, Buchanan does not only claim that there are good reasons for enhancement, but also that the contrary position—the restrictive view—has the burden of proof to provide us with good reasons why enhancement should be morally prohibited or legally regulated. As long as the permissive views are not able to do that, the default status is that enhancement should not be restricted. Is that a helpful starter in the debate? Arguably, it is not—also if employed from the opposite direction[320]—when restrictive positions shift the burden of proof. It merely serves to generate a dialectical asymmetry: In the case just mentioned, the proponent of a permissive view merely needs to argue against its critics while the proponent of a restrictive view is in the uncomfortable position of promoting and defending his own arguments against biotechnological enhancement.

---

[317] For an insightful exception cf. Buchanan 2008: 1–34; Douglas 2015.

[318] Cf. section 5.1.1.1 (»Improved welfare«).

[319] Buchanan 2011a: 12.

[320] It is a striking fact that restrictive views also use this strategy occasionally, although not quite as extensive as permissive views. Cf. for an example Leon Kass, who is concerned that human beings could not »really own the transformations nor experience them as genuinely« (Kass 2003: 24). Kass presents his lack of ownership thesis as a phenomenological fact so that he could be interpreted as reading the What-fuss-question of Buchanan in the opposite direction: it is not the restrictive, but the permissive and mandatory view which has the burden of proof to show that there are good reasons *for* enhancement technologies.

Such a situation, though, does not help to identify the reasons that should count in the debate, because it liberates one party from the burden of providing positive arguments. This makes a well-considered practical consideration almost impossible. In order to avoid this impasse, it seems more fruitful to directly address the reasons that speak for and against enhancement technologies and make them more transparent.[321]

6.2.4 Lack of transparency in ethical grounding

Another challenge in the debate has to do with its lack of transparency in its methodological and structural presuppositions. For one, it is not always clear whether an argument is one that draws from consequentialist, deontological, or virtue ethical resources. As already stated, some of the arguments are highly ambiguous in their formulation. For instance, there are arguments present in the discourse which can be linked to at least two different traditions (e. g. complicity in 5.2.2.3 and 5.2.2.4, authenticity in 5.1.1.2 and 5.1.2.4, or virtue and human nature in 5.1.1.3 and 5.1.2.5). But being precise about ethical grounding is not only important for its own sake. Particularly, if it comes to practical deliberation, it is important to recognize and reflect one's own ethical presuppositions in order to make a justified, all things considered claim. How should we weigh the different arguments if we do not know what is at stake? Of course, this question also calls for more reflections on the process of practical deliberation itself. Are we better off in justifying our all things considered judgments by matters of coherence, self-evidence, or transcendental deduction? Shall we rely our judgments on the sources of individual intuitions, social consensus, or other sources? These are all difficult and important questions well-known in normative theory and metaethics, but they are addressed only occasionally in the debate on enhancement. In order to make progress, however, it seems not only promising but mandatory to put more thoughts in the grounding as it is currently happening in the debate.

---

[321] Our overviews of the respective supporting arguments in section 5.1.1 (»Supporting arguments«), section 5.2.1 (»Supporting arguments«), and section 5.3.1 (»Supporting arguments«) can be seen as a starting point for such a project since it makes the pro arguments visible and therefore as a result available for practical deliberation processes.

6.3 Final thoughts

Many of the enhancement technologies have the potential to significantly alter human lifeforms. Given the prospects and perils of such changes in our socio-biological setup, it should be clear that we need to be very careful in our practical evaluations. The enhancement debate would profit from future work that

a.) … avoids placeholder debates and identifies the »real battleground« of an argument,
b.) … is transparent about the arguments in use and sensitive to their actual strength and decisiveness,
c.) … engages deeply with normative ethics and metaethics in order to sharpen the arguments and the underlying processes of evaluation.

However, these desiderata should not convey the impression that the current discussion on enhancement is methodically immature. As shown in this volume, the debate took a start with theoretically dense, if politically motivated views and developed into a nuanced web of positions and arguments and presents itself as a place of fruitful exchange between the different protagonists. Nevertheless, it seems obvious that even such an elaborate debate can make further progress. We suggest that the points a.)–c.) should not be regarded as fatal failure, but as work packages for future endeavours. The enhancement debate is, like Harris rightly observed, »one of the most significant areas of bioethical interest in the last twenty years.«[322] Given that, it seems promising to pursue it further and to make the debate even more nuanced and detailed than it already is.

References

Ach, J. S. / Beck, B. / Lüttenberg, B. / Stroop, B. (2018): Neuroenhancement: Worum es geht. Ein kritischer Blick auf die Debatte um Neuro-Enhancement. In: Erny, N. / Herrgen, M. / Schmidt, J. C. (eds.): Die Leistungssteigerung des menschlichen Gehirns. Neuro-Enhancement im interdisziplinären Diskurs. Wiesbaden: Springer VS, 37–56.
Agar, N. (1998): Liberal eugenics. In: Public Affairs Quarterly 12 (2), 137–155.
Agar, N. (2007): Where to transhumanism? In: Hastings Center Report 37 (3), 12–17.
Agar, N. (2013): Why is it possible to enhance moral status and why doing so is wrong? In: Journal of Medical Ethics 39 (2), 67–74.

---

[322] Harris 2010: 102.

Allhoff, F. / Lin, P. / Moor, J. / Weckert, J. (2010): Ethics of human enhancement: 25 questions & answers. In: Studies in Ethics, Law, and Technology 4 (1), 1–49.

Appel, J. M. (2008): When the boss turns pusher: A proposal for employee protections in the age of cosmetic neurology. In: Journal of Medical Ethics 34 (8), 616–618.

Archer, A. (2016): Moral enhancement and those left behind. In: Bioethics 30 (7), 500–510.

Bauer, K. (2018): Cognitive self-enhancement as a duty to oneself: A Kantian perspective. In: The Southern Journal of Philosophy 56 (1), 36–58.

Beck, B. (2015): Conceptual and practical problems of moral enhancement. In: Bioethics 29 (4), 233–240.

Beck, B. / Stroop, B. (2015): A biomedical shortcut to (fraudulent) happiness? An analysis of the notions of well-being and authenticity underlying objections to mood enhancement. In: Søraker, J. H. / van der Rijt, J.-W. / de Boer, J. / Wong, P.-H. / Brey, P. (eds.): Well-being in contemporary society. Cham: Springer International Publishing, 115–134.

Berghmans, R. / ter Meulen, R. / Malizia, A. / Vos, R. (2011): Scientific, ethical, and social issues in mood enhancement. In: Savulescu, J. / ter Meulen, R. / Kahane G. (eds.): Enhancing human capacities. Oxford: Wiley Blackwell, 153–165.

Birnbacher, D. (2012): Die ethische Ambivalenz des Enhancement. In: Quante, M. / Rózsa, E. (eds.): Anthropologie und Technik. München: Wilhelm Fink Verlag, 109–126.

Blumenthal-Barby, J. S. / Burroughs, H. (2012): Seeking better health care outcomes: the ethics of using the »nudge«. In: The American Journal of Bioethics 12 (2), 1–10.

Boldt, J. / Maio, G. (2009): Neuroenhancement. Vom technizistischen Missverständnis geistiger Leistungsfähigkeit. In: Müller, O. / Clausen, J. / Maio, G. (eds.): Das technisierte Gehirn: Neurotechnologien als Herausforderung für Ethik und Anthropologie. Paderborn: Mentis, 383–397.

Bolt, L. L. E. (2007): True to oneself? Broad and narrow ideas on authenticity in the enhancement debate. In: Theoretical medicine and bioethics 28 (4), 285–300.

Boorse, C. (1976): What a theory of mental health should be. In: Journal for the Theory of Social Behaviour 6 (1), 61–84.

Boorse, C. (1977): Health as a theoretical concept. In: Philosophy of Science 44 (4), 542–573.

Bostrom, N. / Ord, T. (2006): The reversal test: Eliminating status quo bias in applied ethics. In: Ethics 116 (4), 656–679.

Bostrom, N. (2008): Why I want to be a posthuman when I grow up. In: Gordijn, B. / Chadwick, R. (eds.): Medical enhancement and posthumanity. Dordrecht: Springer, 107–137.

Bostrom, N. / Cirkovic, M. M. (eds.) (2008): Global catastrophic risks. Oxford: Oxford University Press.

Bostrom, N. / Sandberg, A. (2009): The wisdom of nature: An evolutionary heuristic for human enhancement. In: Savulescu, J. / Bostrom, N. (eds.): Human enhancement. Oxford / New York: Oxford University Press, 375–416.

Brock, D. W. (1998): Enhancements of Human Function: Some Distinctions for Policymakers. In: Parens, E. (ed.): Enhancing human traits. Ethical and social implications. Georgetown, Texas: Georgetown University Press, 48–69.

Bublitz, J. C. / Merkel, R. (2009): Autonomy and authenticity of enhanced personality traits. In: Bioethics 23 (6), 360–374.

Buchanan, A. / Brock, D. W. / Daniels, N. / Wikler, D. (eds.) (2001): From chance to choice. Genetics and justice. Cambridge / New York: Cambridge University Press.

Buchanan, A. (2008): Enhancement and the ethics of development. In: Kennedy Institute of Ethics Journal 18 (1), 1–34.

Buchanan, A. (2009a): Moral status and human enhancement. In: Philosophy & Public Affairs 37 (4), 346–381.

Buchanan, A. (2009b): Human nature and enhancement. In: Bioethics 23 (3), 141–150.

Buchanan, A. (2011a): Better than human. The promise and perils of enhancing ourselves. New York: Oxford University Press.

Buchanan, A. (2011b): Beyond humanity? The ethics of biomedical enhancement. Oxford / New York: Oxford University Press.

Cabrera, L. Y. / Weckert, J. (2012): Human enhancement and communication: on meaning and shared understanding. In: Science and Engineering Ethics 19 (3), 1039–1056.

Cabrera, L. Y. (2015): Rethinking human enhancement. New York: Palgrave Macmillan.

Cabrera, L. Y. (2017): Reframing human enhancement: A population health perspective. In: Frontiers in Sociology 2 (4), 1–5.

Caplan, A. L. (2009): Good, better, or best. In: Savulescu, J. / Bostrom, N. (eds.): Human Enhancement. Oxford / New York: Oxford University Press, 199–209.

Carter, A. / Ambermoon, P. / Hall, W. D. (2011): Drug-induced impulse control disorders: A prospectus for neuroethical analysis. In: Neuroethics 4 (2) (Special Issue: Addiction Neuroscience), 91–102.

Carter, J. A. (2017): Intellectual autonomy, epistemic dependence, and cognitive enhancement. In: Synthese, 1–25.

Cerullo, M. A. (2009): Beyond repugnance: Human enhancement and the President's Council on Bioethics. In: Phillips, J. (ed.): Philosophical Perspectives on Technology and Psychiatry. Oxford: Oxford University Press.

Chadwick, R. (2009): Therapy, enhancement and improvement. In: Gordijn, B. / Chadwick, R. (eds.): Medical Enhancement and Posthumanity. Dordrecht: Springer, 25–37.

Chalmers, D. (2010): The character of consciousness. Oxford: Oxford University Press.

Chatterjee, A. (2004): Cosmetic neurology: The controversy over enhancing movement, mentation, and mood. In: Neurology 63 (6), 968–974.

Cho, M. M. / DeVries, A. C. / Williams, J. R. / Carter, C. S. (1999): The effects of oxytocin and vasopressin on partner preferences in male and female prairie voles (Microtus ochrogaster). In: Behavioral Neuroscience 113 (5), 1071–1079.

Clark, A. / Chalmers, D. (1998): The extended mind. In: Analysis 58 (1), 7–19.

Coady, T. (2009): Playing God. In: Savulescu, J. / Bostrom, N. (eds.): Human Enhancement. Oxford / New York: Oxford University Press, 155–180.

Cosman, M. P. (1983): A feast for Aesculapius: historical diets for asthma and seual pleasure. In: Annual Review of Nutrition 3, 1–33.

Crutchfield, P. (2019): Compulsory moral bioenhancement should be covert. In: Bioethics 33 (1), 112–121.

Daniels, N. / Sabin, J. (1997): Limits to health care: Fair procedures, democratic deliberation, and the legitimacy problem for insurers. In: Philosophy & Public Affairs 26 (4), 303–350.

Daniels, N. (2009): Can anyone really be talking about ethically modifying human nature. In: Savulescu, J. / Bostrom, N. (eds.): Human Enhancement. Oxford / New York: Oxford University Press, 25–42.

DeGrazia, D. (2000): Prozac, enhancement, and self-creation. In: Hastings Center Report 30 (2), 34–40.

DeGrazia, D. (2005): Human identity and bioethics. Cambridge / New York: Cambridge University Press.

DeGrazia, D. (2013): Moral enhancement, freedom, and what we (should) value in moral behaviour. In: Journal of Medical Ethics 40 (6), 1–8.

De Haan, A. / De Pauw, S. / van den Akker, A. / Dekovic, M. / Prinzie, P. (2017): Long-term developmental changes in children's lower order big five personality facets. In: Journal of Personality 85 (5), 616–631.

Dennett, D. (2012). The Mystery of David Chalmers. In: Journal of Consciousness Studies, 19 (1–2), 1–2.

Douglas, T. (2007): Enhancement in sport, and enhancement outside sport. In: Studies in Ethics, Law, and Technology 1 (1).

Douglas, T. (2008): Moral enhancement. In: Journal of Applied Philosophy 25 (3), 228–245.

Douglas, T. (2015): The harms of enhancement and the conclusive reasons view. In: Cambridge Quarterly of Healthcare Ethics 24 (1), 23–36.

Earp, B. D. / Wudarczyk, O. A. / Sandberg, A. / Savulescu, J. (2013): If I could just stop loving you: Anti-love biotechnology and the ethics of a chemical breakup. In: The American Journal of Bioethics 13 (11), 3–17.

Elliott, C. (1998): The tyranny of happiness: Ethics and cosmetic psychopharmacology. In: Parens, E. (ed.): Enhancing human traits. Ethical and social implications. Washington D.C.: Norton, 177–188.

Elliott, C. (2003): Better than well: American medicine meets the American dream. New York: Norton.

Erler, A. (2012): One man's authenticity is another man's betrayal: A reply to Levy. In: Journal of Applied Philosophy 29 (3), 257–265.

Erler, A. (2014): Authenticity. In: Bioethics. Rev. 4th ed. Ed. by Bruce Jennings. Farmington Hills, Michigan: Macmillan Reference USA.

Farah, M. J. / Illes, J. / Cook-Deegan, R. / Gardner, H. / Kandel, E./ King, P. / Parens, E. / Sahakian, B. / Wolpe, P. R. (2004): Neurocognitive enhancement: What can we do and what should we do? In: Nature Reviews Neuroscience 5 (5), 421–425.

Foddy, B. / Savulescu, J. (2007): Ethics of performance enhancement in sport: Drugs and gene doping. In: Ashcroft, R. E. / Dawson, A. / Draper, H. / McMillan, J. R. (eds.): Principles of health care ethics. London: John Wiley and Sons, 511–520.

Friele, M. B. (2000): Moralische Komplizität in der medizinischen Forschung und Praxis. In: Wiesing, U. / Simon, A. / von Engelhardt, D. (eds.): Ethik in der medizinischen Forschung. Stuttgart: Schattauer Verlag, 126–136.

Friele, M. B. (2008): Legitimising prohibitive claims in bioethics. In: Newsletter Europäische Akademie 81, 1–3.

Fröding, B. E. (2011): Cognitive enhancement, virtue ethics and the good life. In: Neuroethics 4, 223–234.

Fukuyama, F. (2002): Our posthuman future: Consequences of the biotechnology revolution. New York: Farrar Straus & Giroux.

Galert, T. / Bublitz, J. C. / Heuser, I. / Merkel, R. / Repantis, D. / Schöne-Seifert, B. / Talbot, D. (2009): Das optimierte Gehirn. In: Gehirn & Geist 11, 40–48.

Gazzaniga, M. (2005): The ethical brain. Washington D.C.: Dana Press.

Giubilini, A. / Sanyal, S. (2015): The ethics of human enhancement. In: Philosophy Compass 10 (4), 233–243.

Glannon, W. (2002): Identity, prudential concern, and extended lives. In: Bioethics 16 (3), 266–283.

Green, R. M. (2010): The President's Council on Bioethics – requiescat in pace. In: Journal of Religious Ethics 38 (2), 197–218.

Groll, D. / Lott, M. (2015): Is there a role for »human nature« in debates about human enhancement? In: Philosophy 90 (4), 623–651.

Guillén, M. F. / Suárez, S. L. (2005): Explaining the global digital divide: Economic, political and sociological drivers of cross-national internet use. In: Social Forces 84 (2), 681–708.

Gyngell, C. (2012): Enhancing the species: Genetic engineering technologies and human persistence. In: Philosophy & Technology 25 (4), 495–512.

Habermas, J. (2003): The Future of Human Nature. Cambridge: Polity Press.

Harris, J. (1992): Wonderwoman and superman. The ethics of human biotechnology. Oxford / New York: Oxford University Press.

Harris, J. (2007): Enhancing evolution: the ethical case for making better people. Princeton, New Jersey: Princeton University Press.

Harris, J. (2011): Moral enhancement and freedom. In: Bioethics 25 (2), 102–111.

Hauskeller, M. (2011): Human enhancement and the giftedness of life. In: Philosophical Papers 40 (1), 55–79.

Haverkamp, F. / Ranke, M. B. (1999): The ethical dilemma of growth hormone treatment of short stature: a scientific theoretical approach. In: Hormone Research 51 (6), 301–304.

Heilinger, J.-C. (2010): Anthropologie und Ethik des Enhancements. Berlin / New York: de Gruyter.

Heinrichs, J.-H. (2012): The Sensitivity of Neuroimaging Data. In: Neuroethics 5 (2): 185–195.

Heinrichs, J.-H. (2017): Enhancement: Ein Begriff zwischen Definitionshoheiten? In: Jahrbuch für Wissenschaft und Ethik 21 (1), 69–98.

Heinrichs, J.-H. / Stake, M. (2018): Enhancement: Consequentialist arguments. In: Zeitschrift für Ethik und Moralphilosophie 1 (2), 321–342.

Heinrichs, J.-H. / Stake, M. (2019): Human enhancement: Arguments from virtue ethics. In: Zeitschrift für Ethik und Moralphilosophie 2 (2), 355–373.

Herodotus (2013): The histories. The complete translation, backgrounds, commentaries. Ed. by Jennifer Tolbert Roberts. New York: W. W. Norton & Co.

Holt, R. I. G. / Erotokritou-Mulligan, I. / Sönksen, P. H. (2009): The history of doping and growth hormone abuse in sport. In: Growth Hormone & IGF Research 19 (4), 320–326.

Hursthouse, R. (1996): Normative virtue ethics. In: Crisp, R. (ed.): How should one live? Essays on the virtues. Oxford: Clarendon Press, 19–36.

Hursthouse, R. / Pettigrove, G. (2016): Virtue ethics. In: The Stanford Encyclopedia of Philosophy (Winter 2016 Edition), ed. by Edward N. Zalta, URL https://plato.stanford.edu/archives/win2016/entries/ethics-virtue/ [30 November 2021].

Illes, J. / Gallo, M. / Kirschen, M. P. (2006): An ethics perspective on transcranial magnetic stimulation (TMS) and human neuromodulation. In: Behavioural Neurology 17 (3–4): 149–157.

Illes, J. (ed.) (2017): Neuroethics: Anticipating the Future. Oxford University Press.

Illes, J. (ed.) (2006): Neuroethics: defining the issues in theory, practice, and policy. Oxford: Oxford University Press.

Ilieva, I. / Boland, J. / Farah, M. J. (2013): Objective and subjective cognitive enhancing effects of mixed amphetamine salts in healthy people. In: Neuropharmacology 64, 496–505.

Insel, T. R. / Hulihan, T. J. (1995): A gender-specific mechanism for pair bonding: Oxytocin and partner preference formation in monogamous voles. In: Behavioral Neuroscience 109 (4), 782–789.

Jotterand, F. (2011): »Virtue engineering« and moral agency: Will post-humans still need the virtues? In: AJOB Neuroscience 2 (4), 3–9.

Juengst, E. T. (1998): What does enhancement mean? In: Parens, E. (ed.): Enhancing human traits. Ethical and social implications. Georgetown, Texas: Georgetown University Press, 29–47.

Kahane, G. (2011): Reasons to feel, reasons to take pills. In: Savulescu, J. / ter Meulen, R. / Kahane, G. (eds.): Enhancing human capacities. Oxford: Wiley Blackwell, 166–178.

Kass, L. (2003): Ageless bodies, happy souls: Biotechnology and the pursuit of perfection. In: The New Atlantis 1, 9–28.

Kayser, B. / Mauron, A. / Miah, A. (2005): Legalisation of performance-enhancing drugs. In: The Lancet 366, 21.

King, L. A. (2013): Legal classification of novel psychoactive substances: An international comparison. In: Dargan, P. I. / Wood, D. M. (eds.): Novel Psychoactive Substances. Boston: Academic Press, 3–27.

Kipke, R. (2013): Das »gute Leben« in der Bioethik. In: Ethik in der Medizin 25 (2), 115–128.

Kirsh, D. / Maglio, P. P. (1994): On Distinguishing Epistemic from Pragmatic Action. In: Cognitive Science 18 (4), 513–549

Knell, S. (2015): Die Eroberung der Zeit: Grundzüge einer Philosophie verlängerter Lebensspannen. Berlin: Suhrkamp.

Kramer, P. D. (1994): Listening to Prozac. London: Fourth Estate.

Kraemer, F. (2011): Authenticity anyone? The enhancement of emotions via neuropharmacology. In: Neuroethics 4 (1), 51–64.

Kurzweil, R. (2005): The singularity is near: When humans transcend biology. New York: Viking.

Lattman, P. (2007): The origins of Justice Stewart's »I know it when I see it«. In: Wall Street Journal (September 27, 2007). Law Blog at The Wall Street Journal Online. URL https://blogs.wsj.com/law/2007/09/27/the-origins-of-justice-stewarts-i-know-it-when-i-see-it/ [30 November 2021].

Lavazza, A. (2018a): Memory-Modulation: Self-improvement or self-depletion? In: Frontiers in Psychology 9: 469.

Lavazza, A. (2018b): Cognitive enhancement through genetic editing: A new frontier to explore (and to regulate)? In: Journal of Cognitive Enhancement 2 (4), 388–396.

Lee, P. / George, R. (2008): The nature and basis of human dignity. In: The President's Council on Bioethics (ed.): Human dignity and bioethics. Washington D.C.: US Govt Printing Office, 409–433.

Levy, N. (2007): Rethinking neuroethics in the light of the extended mind thesis. In: American Journal of Bioethics 7 (9), 3–11.

Levy, N. (2011): Neuroethics and the Extended Mind. In: Illes, J. / Sahakian, B. (eds.): Oxford Handbook of Neuroethics. Oxford / New York: Oxford University Press, 285–294.

Levy, N. (2013): There may be costs to failing to enhance, as well as to enhancing. In: American Journal of Bioethics 13 (7), 38–39

Lewens, T. (2012): Human nature: the very idea. In: Philosophy and Technology 25 (4), 459–474.

Liao, S. M. / Sandberg, Anders (2008): The normativity of memory modification. In: Neuroethics 1 (2), 85–99.

Liao, S. M. / Roache, R. (2011): After Prozac. In: Savulescu, J. / ter Meulen, R. / Kahane, G. (eds.): Enhancing Human Capacities. Oxford: Wiley-Blackwell, 245–256.

Lieb, K. (2010): Hirndoping. Warum wir nicht alles schlucken sollten. Mannheim: Artemis & Winkler.

Lin, P. / Mehlman, M. J. / Abney, K. / Galliott, J. (2014): Super soldiers (part 1): What is military human enhancement? In: Thompson, S. J. (ed.): Global issues and ethical considerations in human enhancement technologies. Hershey, Pennsylvania: IGI Global, 119–138.

Little, M. O. (1998): Cosmetic surgery, suspect norms, and the ethics of complicity. In: Parens, E. (ed.): Enhancing human traits: ethical and social implications. Washington D.C.: Georgetown University Press, 162–176.

Lustig, A. (2008): Enhancement technologies and the person: Christian perspectives. In: The Journal of Law, Medicine & Ethics 36 (1), 41–50.

MacIntyre, A. (2007): After virtues. 3. Ed. Notre Dame, Indiana: University of Notre Dame Press.

Macklin, R. (2006): The new conservatives in bioethics: Who are they and what do they seek? In: Hastings Center Report 36 (1), 34–43.

Maier, L. J. / Ferris, J. A. / Winstock, A. R. (2018): Pharmacological cognitive enhancement among non-ADHD individuals. A cross-sectional study in 15 countries. In: International Journal of Drug Policy 58, 104–112.

Maslen, H. / Douglas, T. / Cohen Kadosh, R. / Levy, N. / Savulescu, J. (2015): The regulation of cognitive enhancement devices: Refining Maslen et al.'s model. In: Journal of Law and the Biosciences 2 (3), 754–767.

McMahan, J. (2009): Cognitive disability and cognitive enhancement. In: Metaphilosophy 40 (3–4), 582–605.

Mehlman, M. J. / Lin, P. / Abney, K. (2013): Enhanced warfighters: risk, ethics, and policy. In: Case Legal Studies Research Paper No. 2013-2. URL https://dx.doi.org/10.2139/ssrn.2202982 [30 November 2021].

Meilaender, G. (2008): Human dignity: Exploring and explicating the Council's vision. In: The President's Council on Bioethics (ed.): Human dignity and bioethics. Washington D.C.: US Govt Printing Office, 253–377.

Miah, A. (2011): Ethics issues raised by human enhancement. In: Values and Ethics for the 21st Century. Madrid: BBVA. URL https://www.bbvaopenmind.com/en/articles/ethics-issues-raised-by-human-enhancement/ [30 November 2021].

Mill, J. S. (1969): The collected works of John Stuart Mill. Vol. X. Essays on ethics, religion, and society. Ed. by J. Robson. Toronto: University of Toronto Press.

Moesgen, D. / Klein, M. (2015): Neuroenhancement. Stuttgart: Kohlhammer.

More, M. (2013): The philosophy of transhumanism. In: More, M. / Vita-More, N. (eds.): The transhumanist reader: classical and contemporary essays on science, technology, and philosophy of the human future. Chichester: Wiley-Blackwell, 1–17.

Morrison, M. (2015): Growth hormone, enhancement and the pharmaceuticalisation of short stature. In: Social Science & Medicine 131, 305–312.

Müller, C. P. / Schumann, G. (2011): Drugs as instruments: A new framework for non-addictive psychoactive drug use. In: Behavioral and Brain Sciences 34 (6), 293–310.

Munthe, C. (2019): The black hole challenge: precaution, existential risks and the problem of knowledge gaps. In: Ethics, Policy & Environment 22 (1), 49–60.

Nagel, T. (1974): What is it like to be a bat? In: The Philosophical Review 83 (4), 435–450.

Nyholm, S. / O'Neill, E. (2016): Deep brain stimulation, continuity over time, and the true self. In: Cambridge Quarterly of Healthcare Ethics 25 (4), 647–658.

Nyholm, S. / O'Neill, E. (2017): Deep brain stimulation, authenticity and value: Further reflections. In: Cambridge Quarterly of Healthcare Ethics 26 (4), 658–670.

Olthof, B. / Peeters, A. / Schelle, K. / Haselager, P. (2013): If you're smart, we'll make you smarter. Applying the reasoning behind the development of honours programmes to other forms of cognitive enhancement. In: Lucivero, F. / Vedder, A. (eds.): Beyond therapy v. enhancement? Multidisciplinary analyses of a heated debate. Pisa: Pisa University Press, 117–142.

Orlebeke Caldera, E. (2008): Cognitive enhancement and theories of justice: Contemplating the malleability of nature and self. In: Journal of Evolution and Technology 18 (1), 116–123.

Orr, R. D. (2007): The role of moral complicity in issues of conscience. In: American Journal of Bioethics 7 (12), 23–24.

Parens, E. (1998a): Is Better Always Good? The enhancement project. In: Hastings Center Report 28 (1), 1–17.

Parens, E. (ed.) (1998b): Enhancing human traits. Ethical and social implications. Georgetown, Texas: Georgetown University Press.

Parens, E. (2005): Authenticity and ambivalence. In: Hastings Center Report 35 (5), 34–41.

Persson, I. / Savulescu, J. (2008): The perils of cognitive enhancement and the urgent imperative to enhance the moral character of humanity. In: Journal of Applied Philosophy 25 (3), 162–177.

Persson, I. / Savulescu, J. (2012): Unfit for the future. The need for moral enhancement. Oxford: Oxford University Press.

Persson, I. / Savulescu, J. (2014): Should moral bioenhancement be compulsory? Reply to Vojin Rakic. In: Journal of Medical Ethics 40 (4), 251–252.

Phoenix, C. / Treder, M. (2008). Nanotechnology as global catastrophic risk. In: Bostrom, N. / Cirkovic, M. M. (eds.): Global catastrophic risks. Oxford: Oxford University Press, 481–503.

President's Council on Bioethics (U.S.) (2003): Beyond Therapy: Biotechnology and the Pursuit of Happiness. Washington D.C.: The President's Council on Bioethics.

Prusak, B. G. (2005): Rethinking »liberal eugenics«: Reflections and questions on Habermas on bioethics. In: Hastings Center Report 35 (6), 31–42.

Pugh, J. (2015): Autonomy, natality and freedom: A liberal re-examination of Habermas in the enhancement debate. In: Bioethics 29 (3), 142–152.

Pugh, J. / Kahane, G. / Savulescu, J. (2016): Bioconservatism, partiality, and the human-nature objection to enhancement. In: The Monist 99 (4), 406–422.

Pugh, J. / Maslen, H. / Savulescu, J. (2017): Deep brain stimulation, authenticity and value. In: Cambridge Quarterly of Healthcare Ethics 26 (4), 640–657.

Radoilska, L. (2010): An Aristotelian approach to cognitive enhancement. In: Journal of Value Inquiry 44, 365–375.

Rakic, V. (2014): Voluntary moral bioenhancement is a solution to Sparrow's concerns. In: The American Journal of Bioethics 14 (4), 37–38.

Rakic, V. (2015): We must create beings with moral standing superior to our own. In: Cambridge Quarterly of Healthcare Ethics 24 (1), 58–65.

Rakic, V. (2017): Compulsory administration of oxytocin does not result in genuine moral enhancement. In: Medicine, Health Care and Philosophy 20 (3), 291–297.

Ravelingien, A. / Braeckman, J. / Crevits, L. / De Ridder, D. / Mortier, E. (2009): »Cosmetic neurology« and the moral complicity argument. In: Neuroethics 2 (3), 151–162.

Rawls, J. (1971): A theory of justice. Cambridge, Massachusetts: The Belknap Press of Harvard University Press.

Repantis, D. / Schlattmann, P. / Laisney, O. / Heuser, I. (2009): Antidepressants for neuroenhancement in healthy individuals: a systematic review. In: Poiesis and Praxis 6 (3–4), 139–174.

Repantis, D. / Laisney, O. / Heuser, I. (2010): Acetylcholinesterase inhibitors and memantine for neuroenhancement in healthy individuals: a systematic review. In: Pharmacological Research 61 (6), 473–481.

Repantis, D. / Schlattmann, P. / Laisney, O. / Heuser, I. (2010): Modafinil and methylphenidate for neuroenhancement in healthy individuals: a systematic review. In: Pharmacological Research 62 (3), 187–206.

Rose, S. (2005): The future of the brain. Oxford: Oxford University Press.

Rudman, D. / Feller, A. G. / Nagraj, H. S. / Gergans, G. A. / Lalitha, P. Y. / Goldberg, A. F. / Schlenker, R. A. / Cohn, L. / Rudman, I. W. / Mattson, D. E. (1990): Effects of human growth hormone in men over 60 years old. In: New England Journal of Medicine 323 (1), 1–6.

Rüther, M. / Heinrichs, J.-H. (2019): Human enhancement: Deontological arguments. In: Zeitschrift für Ethik und Moralphilosophie 2, 161–178.

Sandberg, A. (2011): Cognitive enhancement: Upgrading the brain. In: Savulescu, J. / ter Meulen, R. / Kahane G. (eds.): Enhancing human capacities. Oxford: Wiley Blackwell, 71–91.

Sandberg, A. / Fabiano, J. (2017): Modeling the Social dynamics of moral enhancement: Social strategies sold over the counter and the stability of society. In: Cambridge Quarterly of Healthcare Ethics 26 (3), 431–445.

Sandel, M. (2007): The case against perfection. Cambridge, Massachusetts / London: Harvard University Press.

Sandel, M. (2012): The case against perfection: What's wrong with designer children, bionic athletes, and genetic engineering? In: Holland, S. (ed.): Arguing About Bioethics. New York: Routledge, 93–104.

Savulescu, J. / Foddy, B. / Clayton, M. L. (2004): Why we should allow performance enhancing drugs in sport. In: British Journal of Sports Medicine 38 (6), 666–670.

Savulescu, J. / Sandberg, A. (2008): Neuroenhancement of love and marriage: The chemicals between us. In: Neuroethics 1 (1), 31–44.

Savulescu, J. / Sandberg, A. / Kahane, G. (2011): Well-being and enhancement. In: Savulescu, J. / ter Meulen, R. / Kahane, G. (eds.): Enhancing human capacities. Oxford: Wiley-Blackwell, 3–18.

Savulescu, J. / ter Meulen, R. / Kahane, G. (2011): Enhancing human capacities. Oxford: Wiley-Blackwell.

Schermer, M. (2008): On the argument that enhancement is »cheating«. In: Journal of Medical Ethics 34 (2), 85–88.

Schermer, M. / Bolt, I. / de Jongh, R. / Olivier, B. (2009): The future of psychopharmacological enhancements: Expectations and policies. In: Neuroethics 2 (2), 75–87.

Schleim, S. / Quednow, B. B. (2018): How realistic are the scientific assumptions of the neuroenhancement debate? Assessing the pharmacological optimism and neuroenhancement prevalence hypotheses. In: Frontiers in Pharmacology 9 (3), 1–7.

Schramme, T. (2017): Classic concepts of disease. In: International Encyclopedia of Public Health. Ed. by S. R. Quah. Oxford: Academic Press, 44–50.

Searle, J. (1980): Minds, brains, and programs. In: Behavioral and Brain Sciences 3 (3), 417–457.

Shapiro, L. A. (2011): Embodied cognition. New York: Routledge.

Shoemaker, D. (2011): Attributability, answerability, and accountability: Toward a wider theory of moral responsibility. In: Ethics, 121 (3), 602–632.

Siep, L. (2003): Normative aspects of the human body. In: Journal of Medicine and Philosophy 28 (2), 171–185.

Siep, L. (2004): Konkrete Ethik. Grundlagen der Natur- und Kulturethik. Frankfurt a. M.: Suhrkamp.

Silver, L. M. (1997): Remaking Eden. How genetic engineering and cloning will transform the American family. New York: Avon Books.

Silvers, A. (1998): A fatal attraction to normalizing: Treating disabilities as deviations from »species-typical« functioning. In: Parens, E. (ed.): Enhancing human traits: Ethical and social implications. Washington D.C.: Georgetown University Press, 95–123.

Smith, M. E. / Farah, M. J. (2011): Are prescription stimulants »smart pills«? The epidemiology and cognitive neuroscience of prescription stimulant use by normal healthy individuals. In: Psychological Bulletin 137 (5), 717–741.

Sparrow, R. J. (2013): The perils of post-persons. In: Journal of Medical Ethics 39 (2), 80–81.

Sparrow, R. J. (2014): Better living through chemistry? A reply to Savulescu and Persson on »Moral Enhancement«. In: Journal of Applied Philosophy 31 (1), 23–32.

Sturma, D. (2019): Subjekt sein: Über Selbstbewusstsein, Selbstbestimmung und Enhancement. In: Viertbauer, K. / Kögerler, R. (eds.): Neuroenhancement: Die philosophische Debatte. Frankfurt a. M.: Suhrkamp, 115–147.

Synofzik, M. / Schlaepfer, T. E. (2008): Stimulating personality: Ethical criteria for deep brain stimulation in psychiatric patients and for enhancement purposes. In: Biotechnology Journal 3 (12), 1511–1520.

Taylor, C. (1991): The ethics of authenticity. Cambridge, Massachusetts: Harvard University Press.

ter Meulen, R. (2019): Enhancement, hybris, and solidarity: a critical analysis of Sandel's »The case against perfection«. In: Medicine, Health Care and Philosophy 22, 397–405.

The Journal of Law, Medicine & Ethics (2008). Special Issue 36/1. URL https:// journals.sagepub.com/toc/lmec/36/1 [30 November 2021].

Vieth, A. (2010): Neuroenhancement. Zwischen Selbstmanipulation und Manipulation des Selbst. In: Schreiber, J. / Förster, J. / Westermann, S. (eds.): Auf der Suche nach Antworten. 20 Jahre Forum Medizin & Ethik. Münster: Lit, 15–28. Quoted from online version: URL https://www.uni-due.de/imperia/md/content/philosophie/ vieth/materialien/neuroenhancement_selbstmanipulation_manipulation_des_ selbst_vi.pdf [30 November], 1–15.

Wada (2020): World Anti-Doping Agency. URL www.wada-ama.org [30 November 2021].

Walsh, P. J. (2017): Cognitive extension, enhancement, and the phenomenology of thinking. In: Phenomenology and the Cognitive Sciences 16 (1), 33–51.

Wasserman, D. / Liao, S. M. (2008): Issues in the pharmacological induction of emotions. In: Journal of Applied Philosophy 25 (3), 178–192.

Wasserman, D. (2014): When bad people do good things: Will moral enhancement make the world a better place? In: Journal of Medical Ethics 40 (6), 374–375.

Wikler, D. (1979): Paternalism and the mildly retarded. In: Philosophy & Public Affairs 8 (4), 377–392.

Wikler, D. (2009): Paternalism in the age of cognitive enhancement: Do civil liberties presuppose roughly equal mental ability? In: Savulescu, J. / Bostrom, N. (eds.): Human enhancement. Oxford / New York: Oxford University Press, 341–355.

Wittgenstein, L. (1999): Philosophical Investigations, G. E. M. Anscombe and R. Rhees (eds.). Oxford: Blackwell.

Yudkowsky, E. (2008): Artificial intelligence as a positive and negative factor in global risk. In: Bostrom, N. / Cirkovic, M. M. (eds.): Global catastrophic risks. Oxford: Oxford University Press, 303–345.

Contact Details

Jan-Hendrik Heinrichs, PD Dr. phil., Research Associate at the Institute of Ethics in the Neurosciences (INM-8) at the Forschungszentrum Jülich (FZJ). Contact: Ethics in the Neurosciences (INM-8), Forschungszentrum Jülich, 52425 Jülich. URL http://www.fz-juelich.de

Julia Ihde, M.A., Research Associate at the German Reference Centre for Ethics in the Life Sciences (DRZE), University of Bonn. Contact: Bonner Talweg 57, 53113 Bonn. URL http://www.drze.de

Dirk Lanzerath, Prof. Dr. phil., Executive Manager of the German Reference Centre for Ethics in the Life Sciences (DRZE), University of Bonn, as well as Honorary Professor for Ethics and Research Ethics, University of Applied Sciences Bonn-Rhein-Sieg. Contact: Bonner Talweg 57, 53113 Bonn. URL http://www.drze.de

Markus Rüther, PD Dr. phil., Research Associate at the Institute of Ethics in the Neurosciences (INM-8) at the Forschungszentrum Jülich (FZJ). Contact: Ethics in the Neurosciences (INM-8), Forschungszentrum Jülich, 52425 Jülich. URL http://www.fz-juelich.de

Mandy Stake, M.A., Research Associate at the Institute of Ethics in the Neurosciences (INM-8) at the Forschungszentrum Jülich (FZJ). Contact: Ethics in the Neurosciences (INM-8), Forschungszentrum Jülich, 52425 Jülich. URL http://www.fz-juelich.de

Dieter Sturma, Prof. Dr. phil., Professor of Philosophy at the University of Bonn, Director of the German Reference Centre for Ethics in the Life Sciences (DRZE) and the Institute for Science and Ethics (IWE), University of Bonn, as well as Director of the Institute of Ethics in the Neurosciences (INM-8) at the Forschungszentrum Jülich (FZJ). Contact: Bonner Talweg 57, 53113 Bonn. URL http://www.dieter-sturma.de